Not in Vain,
A Promise Kept

Not in Vain, A Promise Kept

MELISSA MULLAMPHY

Not in Vain, A Promise Kept

Copyright © 2021 Melissa Mullamphy

ISBN-13 (eBook): 978-1-7348026-6-5
ISNB-13 (Hardcover): 978-1-7348026-2-7
ISBN-13 (Paperback): 978-1-7348026-3-4

CONTENTS

DEDICATION

Medical professionals will diagnose you at some point in your life. They will arrive at that diagnosis using clues on what they see, your medical history, testing, their knowledge of medicine, and your description of symptoms.

They will compile a list of what your illness could be and eliminate the clues that do not fit.

What is left will be your diagnosis.

The next step will be to discuss possible treatment options. But an empowered, liberated and confident patient will ask, "What else can it be?" You have the right to question them. Not everyone fits nicely into the case studies and tests.

Did they get it all?

Were you honest with your history?

Were they really listening, or was it a quick appointment? Was the medical team consistent? Did they write everything down? Did you ask them what their experience was with your diagnosis? Did the medical provider's behavior convince you that they were interested in your case, or did you feel rushed and that you were just another ten-minute time slot?

For the most part, the problem is not bad people in healthcare: it is that good people are working in a lousy system that needs to be made safer with more checks and balances, communication, empathy, and oversight. Patients, family members, and advocates need to recognize and have the confidence to fight, question everything, and double-check on decisions made by those in charge. When you are sick, you feel like you have lost control.

That is why you are the patient.

The reality is you do have some control, just as those who advocate for you do. Let them help you; you do not have to go it alone.

This book is dedicated to all the patients, families, loved ones, friends, nurses, doctors, lab technicians, x-ray technicians, aids, and everyone who finds themselves either working in or needing help from an imperfect system.

In Loving Memory of my mom,
Constance E. Burns

Special thanks to my family and friends for putting up with me over the last ten years, through my grief, anger, and depression. I have had many false starts and a lot of project creep, but I genuinely feel that the time that passed, and, with it, the healing, gave me a better ability to share more and fine-tune my message for this memoir. I know I have not been easy to deal with since December 4, 2010, and will be forever changed, but you have stuck with me through it and never gave up on me. Taking on something like this is not easy, as my mom had about two inches of medical records, and I wrote about five versions during various points of the past ten years, making the words and tone based on where my headspace was at the time. While this type of writing can be very therapeutic, it caused me to relive some of my life's worst times. To Anthony and Luke, especially, I thank you for allowing me the time and patience to fulfill this promise to my mother, and I hope it will make you proud.

INTRODUCTION

"If I cannot move heaven, I will raise hell."
Virgil, *The Aeneid*

In life you will run into many challenges that you'll have to decide how to handle. Some will be layups, and others will test you both emotionally and physically, sometimes to the point where you will question your own sanity and ability to keep going. You will run into people who will help you through life's trials, and others who will be content to sit back and watch you implode. When you're in a crisis, you'll know pretty quickly which friends and family members actually give a fuck and which do not. It's an unfortunate reality, but sooner or later, you will understand that most of the time you are traveling solo in the journey of life. As they say, you come into this world alone, and you go out of this world alone.

You must learn to trust your own instincts; you do not need anyone else's seal of approval. Often, with crisis comes conflict. You will have to face hostility and opposition. You have to stay the course and face the collisions head on. This book tells the story of my family and myself facing a daily battle during my mom's eight-month fight with ovarian cancer. We worked together as a well-greased machine, but almost every day, we had a fight on our hands. Sometimes, it was an internal battle, as we helped my mom manage her illness and supported her in the fight of her life, and other times it was an external one, as we confronted the healthcare system, hospital staff, and endless bureaucracy.

So, why am I writing this book? During one of the more frustrating moments of our eight-month journey, when my mom and I were alone on the cardiology floor, she said to me, "Melissa, don't ever be stupid like me." She meant that I should go to the doctor, get regular check-ups, and take good care of myself so I didn't find myself in the same position she was in. It is common for people living with cancer to experience guilt. Guilt is usually based on the patient's feelings of "what ifs." My mom knew she was very sick and had probably had about six months of symptoms that she had either self-treated. She was just too scared to go see a doctor sooner. In came the guilt and self-doubt. She never wanted to be a burden to anyone.

You will read later in this book that we, as a family, were put through the wringer with her care and had to oversee everything ourselves. I didn't realize it then, but life was about to throw us a hard and fast curveball. A ball that, no matter how talented the batter and how the team stuck to the game strategy to win, was going to put the MVP of our family in a fight for her life. I promised her that night that somehow, some way, the world was going to know what was happening to her. Little did I know what was ahead, but I kept my promise, and she did not die in vain.

I want you, the reader of this book, to learn to advocate for your loved ones. Learn what I learned. Understand your rights and how to navigate the healthcare system. It is not one size fits all, and it is only becoming more complex, as healthcare is a political football right now. Use your voice, and remember that you are not there to make friends. Sometimes you have to be the biggest mouth in the room, but speaking up can save your loved one's life.

Sometimes you have to be an insufferable asshole to get things done. Trust me when I tell you that. You have to wear many hats. One day you may have to be an "acting" nurse, doctor, researcher, politician, lawyer, salesperson, aid, student, psychologist, planner, and most importantly, an advocate. The list is endless. Your goal is not clear all of the time, but you must have the courage to fight the good fight and celebrate the little wins. You also have to accept the losses and defeats. Look around the waiting room in any hospital or clinic, and you will see people waiting to hear good news. You can see it on their faces: the worry, anxiety, and uncertainty. We all go through it.

My hope is that through sharing Mom's story, it may better your game and help you have more wins than losses. If nothing else, I want to help you know your rights and your loved one's rights and give you a couple tips that I learned along the way. If sharing my years as a fuck-up suffering from grief, PTSD, anger, and depression while self-medicating to repress my feelings can help someone understand that grief is not cut and dry, or black and white, that there is no right way of doing it, that you shouldn't be like me but should seek appropriate help instead, then I have accomplished what I set out to do. If what we learned the hard way through Mom's eight -month battle helps one person ask that tough question and go up the chain of command, then my job is done, and I am grateful. Bringing awareness and insight to others may mean that Mom's suffering was not in vain. Perhaps your loved one will still suffer anger, depression, or worse, death, because as the doctors told us on day one, cancer is not a "friendly" disease. But you will have tried your best and maybe learned some tips for the shit game you are about to play.

Dealing with the healthcare system can be a matter of life or death. I'm not saying that all medical and hospital staff and organizations are to be feared. I'm not saying all doctors make gross errors. Of course, they are human, and we all make mistakes. I'm not saying you can't trust what a professional tells you. But you need to be there, you need to ask the tough questions, you need to take notes, you need to watch over your loved one and advocate for them when they cannot or won't. They are overwhelmed and emotional. They are scared. As you will read in my experience, this role is not a choice you will have. If someone does not step up and take on the role or roles bad things can happen. I can almost guarantee it.

Things will get overlooked, and that will only compound the mental and physical suffering your loved one is going through. There are millions of potential reasons malpractice happens. It could be as simple as the healthcare provider having a bad day or too big a caseload. It could be pure and honest human error. They *could* just be fucking lazy and not give a shit. Some doctors might have been in the game too long and are not open and educated in new treatment protocols.

The **Hippocratic Oath** is a sworn agreement made by physicians when they become doctors. It includes a promise to share knowledge, to help the ill and *not cause harm*, and to never give a deadly drug or help another to use one.

All of the healthcare facilities and any medical staff in this book have been given aliases to protect their anonymity.

If they get their hands on this book, they will remember and know who they are. It is an unforgettable case. That is okay with me. There is no fiction here. It's real, raw, and necessary to be told.

Some have asked, "How do you get over it?" "How do you forgive?" "How do you go on?" For me, you don't get over it. You learn to exist without the one you lost. How do you forgive the mistakes made as loved ones suffer? You don't. At least, I don't. I still hold on to the anger toward those who made a sick lady sicker, a suffering lady suffer more, a dying woman go through every possible side effect and consequence of cancer that was possible. You go on because you have to. Life goes on. Even when you think, *there is no fucking way, I can do this*, you can, and you will.

Batter up, here goes nothing.

PROLOGUE

A Letter to My Mother:

It will be ten years in December, Ma, and I'm still pretty fucked up about you being gone. You've missed so much. I've needed you so many times, and you were not there. It sucks. I thank God for my husband, Anthony, and my son, Luke, as they are the glue that keeps me together. Anthony was my rock through your illness and passing. He had to pick up the pieces when you died, and I'm afraid he was in over his head when it came to my mental ability to cope with your loss. It hasn't been easy. I'm not the first kid to lose a parent to cancer, and I won't be the last, but the grief is still in my gut and buried in my brain. Every day and night, it haunts me—your passing and what life has become without you.

Sometimes, I'm still angry. I would also say envious, or, at times, resentful of those who still have their moms, even though I know it's wrong. I used to feel too guilty to ever tell anyone that, but the anger and envy would just come over me, and I could not control it. I would get a pit in my stomach, a giant void. I'd hear of people who got cancer and beat it, and say, why not you? I would be happy for them but angry at the same time.

I know it sounds selfish, but it is the truth.

I wish I believed there was a "reason" behind losing you, that I could believe all those platitudes like "God needed you," "It was your time," or my favorite, "Everything happens for a reason," but I can't get my head around any of it. I can't find any reason. I have read books about religion, grief, and the reality of heaven. I even tried to understand Ephesians 1:11: "All things are done according to God's plan and decision, and God chose us to be his own people in union with Christ because of his own purpose, based on what he had decided from the very beginning," but I don't buy it. I have had many very emotional debates about this personally, and I'll never buy it. I can't, I won't.

You didn't do anything wrong. You were always a shining light, even in the darkest of trying times. How can one believe that it is God's plan if a five-year-old dies from cancer or a tragic accident kills a car full of kids because someone is going the wrong way on the highway? I just don't have that mindset. Perhaps it would make life easier, but I doubt I'll ever get there. Trust me, people have tried to convince me, telling me "Your destiny was set the day you were born." But I call bullshit.

I don't pretend to be perfect. I have made plenty of mistakes since you died. I have deep fucking scars that I've learned to live with. For the most part, they are closed now, but the scab is ripped off at random and inconvenient times. It could be a holiday, walking through the greeting card section on Mother's Day, or going home to visit Daddy. It kills me to go there, because even though he has changed some things, you are still everywhere. It took me four years to help Daddy and Alicia clean out your closets, decide what we were keeping, and give the rest to Goodwill. Alicia did the brunt of it, because I was still a walking shit-show. When I go there, I often find myself walking into your bedroom, looking at pictures, and going into your closet or drawers to smell your things. I get lost in your handwriting on the pictures of your grandchildren and other family members taped to your dresser and the list of phone numbers still on the wall in the kitchen, or I just sit in the living room and relive the night you died. I look at the couch, but I rarely sit on it. I see the CD player we played for comfort when you were curled up on the couch trying to hold onto this life. I open it, and the same CD is in it. I look at the blanket you were wrapped in when you died; I can still see the coffee table full of meds and the chair I sat in as I watched your chest rise and fall after we called in hospice.

Reading this aloud, I realize it makes me sound like a nut, but it's the truth. You know that saying? That some "secrets" are meant to be told to the right people? This is my attempt to reach an audience that will recognize some of this behavior and say to themselves, "Sounds about right" or "I'm not the only one," or "I guess everyone handles things differently." There is no "how-to" or "grief guide" to follow, although I have read many. When you first died, I attended grief groups. Yup, I brought myself there even though I "knew it all" and have a master's degree in counseling psychology. I wasn't passing this test. This was different. This was raw. This was my mother. No fucking way. I went for a couple of months, but although I know group therapy works, and I have led many successful group therapy sessions, it was probably too soon. I did not like telling my story each week when a new member joined. It wasn't, "Hi, my name is Melissa, and I'm an alcoholic," it was "Hi, my name is Melissa, and my mom just died from ovarian cancer, and this is how." The same feelings would take over when I left those sessions, anger, sadness, and resentment.

I was very blessed with my employer for the time during your illness and after you passed, particularly during the most hellish period—May 2010 to January 2011. They took excellent care of me. If I needed to leave, I left. If I needed to take time off, they covered me. The man in charge said, "Missy, nobody wants to be in your boat. If you need to leave, leave. If you need to stay home and take care of your family, we will sweep up after you." They gave me a lot of latitude and support, and I will forever be grateful. I wasn't in the work game 100 percent during that time. I was in maybe 50 on a good day. They knew it, and they supported me all the way to the top. When you died, I was able to take short-term disability to get my brain and health together. My company saw the 115-pound, anxious and depressed person who gave no fucks and was in shambles. I was in no condition to be the leader I needed to be. I was angry, had no patience, and I'm embarrassed to say I didn't treat everyone very well, but I was dying inside, mentally and physically. I had to buy size zero and two clothes and layer them, because I was embarrassed by how skinny I was. I had to get my work clothes tailored because a size two was too big; I tried to find corporate gear in the "juniors" sections at Macy's. As someone with a master's in psychology, I knew the criteria for diagnosis and the DSM V (Diagnostic Statistical Manual 5th Edition, used to diagnose psychiatric disorders). I had textbook acute depression, grief, anxiety, and PTSD.

As you know, I also had experience working in psychiatric emergency rooms and step-down houses and ran group therapy sessions. I saw it all, and because of that, I did not seek the proper help. Instead, I self-treated. I knew better, but I was on autopilot trying to manage work, being a decent mom, wife, sister, daughter, and friend while running on empty and existing in total emotional chaos. My mind was still constantly playing back the terrible scene of your last moments on that couch.

I didn't tell anyone that I had flashbacks of your last moments more times a day than I can count until I broke over a year later. The images stopped me from sleeping, hit me when I was driving, sitting at my desk, and any time I was not concentrating, which was a lot. I tried to switch my focus and get the movie out of my head, but it just didn't work. If it did work, it was temporary. I should have taken my employer up on their option to leave, but I felt I owed them because they were so good to me while you were sick. They offered me a leave option many times, in private conversations, with management and friends taking me to the side, trying to convince me to take the time, but I felt it would not be fair as their support was something you don't see anywhere. It just does not happen. I also thought working would fill a void and be a much-needed distraction, but I only pushed all of my grief and anger deeper, to a point of almost no return. It is easier to distract yourself and stay busy, to block the pain with pills, than to deal with what is killing you inside. I had spent the entire year in self-destruct mode, taking anti-depressants and anti-anxiety meds. I knew how they worked, why they worked, all the way down to the part of your brain in which they operate, and during this time, I needed them to function. Funny thing is, I was never a medicine advocate because working in a psychiatric emergency room taught me that one size doesn't fit all; everyone who was discharged from the emergency room left with meds, and I was against that. I also saw their overuse in step-down houses, residential facilities designed to give patients more independence after being in rehab or a mental facility. I felt the medications were handed out too much, and I'd never need them. Boy, was I wrong on that one. It's sometimes easy to judge from a distance, but once you are in the situation, things look very different.

I stopped taking anti-anxiety meds in the summer of 2011. I knew they were a Band-Aid, and I knew I needed to get off them before it was too late. I was playing with fire, because eventually, I would become addicted even though I was taking them as prescribed. The reality is, I could not have a conversation for months after you passed without crying, so it was a necessary evil for me at the time. They allowed me to function, to push on, deal with life, sometimes sleep, deal with the fact that you were never coming back, and I felt cheated. You were only 68.

We all know stress does not help any physical disease you have, and after years of colitis, inflammatory bowel disease, and GI problems, things were bound to worsen even more. I did not eat because I was always nauseated. I think it was anxiety and GI issues combined. So, I continued this vicious cycle of untreated grief, anger, self-destruction, and self-medicating until the colitis kicked in and I bought myself a five day stay in the hospital. I was weak, bleeding, and basically emaciated.

It was bound to happen because I was not taking care of myself. It was the week of Christmas, and the last Christmas sucked because you died on December 4th. I was not going to miss or ruin Luke's second. I actually lied about my symptoms to get discharged. I was on mega doses of steroids and barely sleeping. I had terrible insomnia, depression, and anxiety; add the steroids, and I was a walking zombie. I looked like a corpse. If I slept an hour a night, that was good, and I still worked every day. I commuted and tried to keep a semi-normal routine. Alicia watched Luke, who was my only light and reason to smile.

Anthony's birthday was in January, so I decided to throw him a party. He had endured months of hell from me and taken over the household ship for a long time, and I wanted to do something special for him. I had everything set. We had probably fifty people coming, I was ready to go, and then it happened: I had a grand mal seizure in my living room about thirty minutes before everyone was to arrive. All I remember is waking up on the couch, being held down, and EMTs walking into my living room, removing me, and placing me into an ambulance. I didn't want to go. I didn't want to sit on the couch, and I could not get my head around the fact that I had actually flown into the kitchen, hit my head on the tile, and turned blue. Poor Anthony was a mess, and my nephew was with me, making sure I was breathing. I really had no idea what had happened. I felt fine, and I had no interest in going to the hospital. I was actually pissed off because I had done so much work to prepare for the party. Surprise, surprise— I learned later that it is common to wake up from a seizure and be agitated.

In the emergency room, they drew blood and had me on a monitor. Epilepsy did not run in our family. They assumed medication was the cause. Hell, the way I looked, I would too. I also gave the EMTs the meds in my pocketbook, but they did not realize that I kept them there, and the scripts were full from my discharge before Christmas. But it looked terrible to anyone who was at my house that evening. Toxicology was negative for everything, benzodiazepines, or opiates, which I tried to tell them, but I had to let the process of elimination work. If it looks like a duck and quacks like a duck, it's a duck. For months I was a human traffic accident, and everyone was looking around at the wreckage. The party went on at the house, but my close friends were distraught and rattled. My best friends sat on my porch, helpless and crying. You know who you are, dear friends who remain in my inner circle today. They searched my house while I was at the hospital, looking for medicine. Thankfully, they only found dog pills, antibiotics, GI meds, and vitamins.

Initially, I wasn't happy that they had gone through my stuff, but they were scared, and I got it. I looked like shit. The gas tank was empty, and I weighed 110 pounds with clothes on. If the situation were reversed, I probably would have done the same or staged some form of intervention. I found out later that they were trying to do one. To make a long story short, an MRI found my hippocampus was not balanced, one side is larger than the other, and I was prone to seizures.

They had just decided to come out and play at the age of 41.

Looking back, it was a very distressing time for many of my relationships. People were trying to help, but when you know that you are not taking certain medications and people do not believe you to the point of calling you a liar to your face, you get angry and resentful. For a while, I had Anthony come to my appointments as support, and, quite frankly, an auditor with full HIPAA access. I had a lot of resentment and even invited people to go to the lab with me, to be tested again. I offered to host a lab party; yes, I was bitter. I had some tough conversations and opened up to those closest to me. In hindsight, I know those giving me the most shit did it because they cared, and they were tired of watching me self-destruct. The depression, anxiety, and grief did not go away just because I stopped taking anti- anxiety medication. I just went to a good professional, and, after years of therapy and introspection, I slowly developed better coping mechanisms. While the sadness is still there, I can finally breathe and have a conversation about you without crying. I won't lie, there are times when I still can go off the deep end, but they are isolated incidents, and usually, there is some kind of trigger.

Unfortunately, I hit my head pretty hard during the first grand mal seizure, and I had a couple, which caused a closed head injury and cognitive damage. My main symptom of the head injury was memory loss. I was actually scared because I was forgetting a lot.

Cognitive issues showed up in my daily life, but particularly at work. For example, when I was in meetings or conference calls at work, I found myself repeating myself to clients and to my work colleagues. At home, I would repeat myself a lot or get into arguments over whether I had communicated something important or not. It got to the point where I began conversations saying, "Tell me if I told you this already." Everyone knew something was wrong with me, but nobody wanted to say it. I knew too, but I was embarrassed. The MRI showed changes, but due to my age, occupation, and education, they could not figure out this cognitive decline. I think some people actually thought I was making it up. Who the hell would make up being a bumbling idiot? I went from leading meetings with brass and managing staff domestically to attending meetings with an outline or script to ensure that I did not repeat myself or forget anything. I would do simple spreadsheets (copying data from one source to another), and the numbers would not balance, and sometimes it was as if I had dyslexia because they would be transposed. I mean holy shit, who does that? Yes, I was still grieving but I had the world by the balls in my career if I wanted it.

I didn't want it.

I wasn't capable of meeting my role's expectations. I got myself tested for early Alzheimer's because I knew something was wrong—very wrong. I went to a doctor at Burke Rehab, who was also the head injury doctor for the New York Giants. He was very well published on post-concussive syndrome, traumatic brain injury, and cognition. I paid out of pocket for this appointment, and it took about three hours. He also interviewed Anthony.

I distinctly remember his telling me that that day, "You have a severe problem here." He diagnosed me with Cognitive Impairment

NOS. That means there is too much shit to pigeonhole me into a clean diagnosis after many interviews and scans; it was "not otherwise specified."

We ruled out the seizure meds causing cognitive decline, because, trust me: they can make you a walking zombie. I wasn't on other meds, so the problem had to be biological. I stopped working in the corporate world at the end of 2013, just shy of a twenty-year career in reinsurance. After each seizure that you have, you lose your driver's license in New York, so after being out for two long periods and losing a lot of cognitive function, I retired on my terms. Looking back in the rearview, I was very blessed to have such a great employer that supported me for all those years.

I left my role, as you can't lead a team or represent a great company to your clients when you make mistakes. Thankfully, I was able to leave on my own merit and stay home to raise Luke. From the day I found out I was pregnant with Luke until today, he and Anthony have been the saving grace of all my heartaches. His miraculous birth gave me a reason to keep going and be happy. Our party of three with our fur babies is my center, and for that, I am so grateful.

So, ten years later, I'm keeping my promise to you, Ma. I'm getting your story out. Not everyone agrees with me in doing so, but when have I really listened, especially if I was passionate about something as important as this? Some say, "Missy stop living in the past," "Move on," "It's not going to change anything." I've heard it all. I can tell you that the process of writing this, sharing my scars, becoming vulnerable to my grief, self-destruction, being transparent, poring over your medical records and going through this has been a healing journey for me. I'll admit going back sometimes brought me sorrow and anger, but to me, it is worth every emotion if it helps one person.

I won't lie and say it has all been easy for our family since you died, that it has been without strife. But I find nothing in life really worth fighting for is. We all handled your loss differently. I don't believe in the "norms" of grief. I think we are all managing the best we can holding on to beautiful memories that a shit disease cannot take away from us. They say death can bring out the best and worst in families. I think we have held our own. It is a hard lesson to learn that you often do not realize how much you love someone until they are gone. I wish we had made more memories. I wish Luke was able to enjoy you. I wish I had told you I love you more. I wish we had more fucking time. I miss you, Ma.

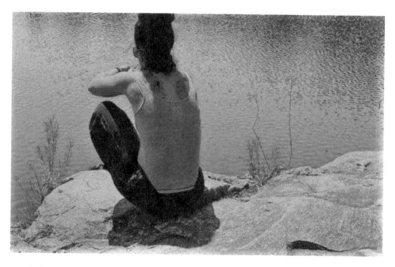

This is me at 115 pounds, riddled with anxiety, depression, and PTSD.
I did not do the grief thing well.

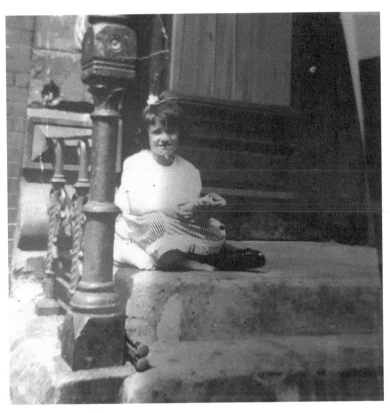

My mom, Brooklyn, NY.

1

WHO WE ARE

Who was Constance E. Burns? Her middle name was Elsa, and she hated it. She was born in 1942, raised Catholic, half-Italian and half-Irish, or so we thought until Ancestry.com told us otherwise. Years ago, I ran my DNA and found out I had French, German, Greek, Welsh and English and American Indian. My mother was the only girl out of five siblings, an extraordinary girl who was only two pounds at birth, back when most babies did not survive that kind of premature delivery. So, Mom was a fighter from the very beginning. My grandmother had pneumonia when she delivered Mom, and both of them almost died. As I remember it from my great-grandmother, the story is she put Mom in a blanket and some sort of oven to keep her warm and alive. During her childhood, Mom had rheumatic fever and was sick a lot. She was close to her brothers, but two lived in other states. Mom lived in Watertown, NY, Brooklyn, NY, White Plains, NY, and eventually Brewster, NY. She was from a generation of strength, not complainers, and she always had great ambition. She was a very proper lady with profound ethical and moral standards. From the day I was born, she worked as a waitress at night, forty years of waiting tables and dealing with the public. Until the evening before we went to the emergency room because Mom had a mystery mass growing in her stomach, she was serving trays of spaghetti and hamburgers to the public, all while carrying around a fifteen-pound tumor in her stomach.

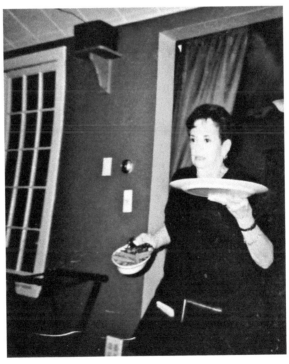

My mom waited tables for 40 years and up until the day before she went to the Emergency Room.

She had the strength of a bull. She would often do yard work; my dad would tell her not to, but she'd do it anyway. The house was always immaculate. She was very creative, a talented artist in many areas, from oil paintings, calligraphy, and ceramics to baking and designing. My father was an operating engineer and would get laid off in the wintertime, so he supplemented his income by plowing, and of course, my mom worked about four nights a week. They made sacrifices when they had to, but my sister and I never wanted for anything. Growing up, we didn't have many extras, but we were spoiled, considering what they had. We call my dad "Mr. Miyagi" because he's so meticulous about taking care of the lawn and everything outside. If there is no work to be done, he will find it or make it.

We lived in a little town an hour outside of Manhattan in Brewster, New York, in a small house of about 900 square feet. When Mom had me, I was breech; it was 1970, and we both almost died, a bit like when her mother gave birth to her. They told Mom and Dad no more kids after me. We lived a pretty healthy blue-collar suburban life. My dad is a character; he can be a little rough around the edges. He's very direct, a man's man, who worked as a volunteer fireman for over fifty years and is still an active member. Because both of our parents had such a strong work ethic, my sister Alicia and I are not afraid of work either. My sister and I had standard household rules, daily chores, and responsibilities.

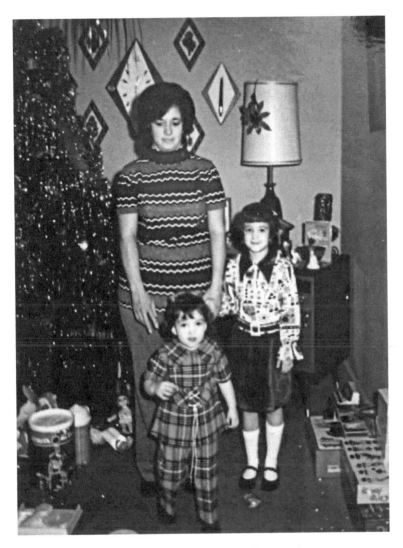

Christmas 1973, My mom, sister Alicia, and me.

such a good waitress many patrons would wait to be placed in "Connie's" section. They only wanted Mom to wait on them. I remember she usually worked on Christmas Eve because it was a big money night, and then when she came home late, she decorated the tree and played Santa Claus. One Christmas, she actually got a real mink coat as a "tip." She remembered the birthdays of her customers, the workers in the kitchen, and all her friends. She was always baking a celebratory cake for somebody.

My mom was a giver in all ways. She always put everyone before herself. I look back now and realize that it is part of why she got so sick. She ignored the symptoms, was afraid to go to the doctor, never gave into the pain, and wanted to keep the train on the tracks. She was the matriarch of our family. She was the glue that kept everything in line, the fulcrum, the strength. She didn't want to show weakness, or, as she put it when she was sick, she didn't want to "burden" anyone. I think her love for us actually worked against her in the end.

My sister is four years older; while we have many similarities, we are also very different. My sister is organized and generally always has a plan; she's a bit more reserved and avoids conflict. I'm more spontaneous, less organized, and a lot like my dad. I don't look for battles, but because I can be very direct, they find me. During stress or a crisis, Alicia and I make a good team and bring balance to each other's strengths and weaknesses. When our mom got sick, she took care of her end, I took care of mine, and we were in constant communication over the phone, email, or text. We always knew what the other was doing.

We were in no way prepared for any of what was ahead. There

were no rules, no "how to's," but we managed as well as we could for the hell we had entered. Trauma makes us all crack. Defeat isn't an option. We were entering a phase of borrowed time, but we did not know it yet. We weren't easily intimidated, and we were in no way going to surrender. But fuck, to this day, I don't know how we made it through. Hope has a way of pushing you even when you are on your fucking knees and just surviving.

2

MAY

The day our journey with this fucked up system began, the eight-month forced march through hospitals and chemotherapy and surgery, was otherwise actually a pretty nice day. My husband and I had just returned from our condo in Myrtle Beach; we were doing the normal back-from-vacation settling in with Luke. Soon after we returned to our house, my mother called me, crying on the other end of the phone. She told me she had a large "bump" on her stomach, that it was growing, and that she knew "it was bad." She had recently watched an episode of Dr. Oz that featured ovarian cancer, and before we ever saw a single doctor, she was convinced that it was cancer.

Initially, I thought it was probably a bowel obstruction that might be serious but fixable. Even though my mom told me she knew it was bad, we had to convince her to go to the emergency room. Unfortunately, both of my parents avoided doctors. It was the generation, and, as they say, once you are married a long time, you turn into your spouse. My Dad lived with an incorrect diagnosis of pneumonia for weeks while he filled up with water and did not tell anyone until he went back forcibly to his General Practitioner (GP) and he was in congestive heart failure. Even then knowing he was at risk, they both decided they were going to put off going to Yale to find out what was wrong until after the holidays. It took my father's GP to call the house and tell both of my parents he would be dead in three days if he did not go right away. It is just how they are built. I'm confident my mom self-treated for months before the day we went to the emergency room with the hopes that something would work or this thing growing in her abdomen would somehow disappear. But it didn't, and this is where all of our heartache began.

The resident Emergency Room (ER) physician entered the room, palpated the mass, and looked at my sister and me with concern. My mother continued to say she knew it was terrible; it was cancer. "I saw it on Dr. Oz." The physician ordered a pelvic CAT scan with contrast and had my mother drink barium in preparation for the test. We later learned she had fluid in her abdomen that was so dense it made drinking the barium difficult for her; it took her a long time to finish it all. As a side note, my mom was 147 pounds at this ER visit. I think the ER doctors got a bad vibe because of her age; she was 68, and ovarian cancer often develops in women in their sixties, once menopause is over.

We tried to make it "funny" while she forced this nasty white liquid down. If you've never had it, trust me; it's disgusting. Although the three of us were stricken with fear, we kept telling one another, "Things like this happen all the time; usually, these things are benign," etc. We tried to make light of the situation.

When they took Mom to radiology, my dad arrived and waited with us for the results. He avoids stress at all costs and did not want to believe that it was a big deal. After about two hours, the ER physician returned and asked if he could talk to my parents privately. At that point, all the fears I'd tried to keep in the back of my mind came full circle into reality. My mom's eyes were red, and she was crying.

When she saw my sister and me, she began to cry more. "I knew it. I knew it. I told you!" She had a 23-centimeter mass on her ovary. Yes, read that again. Twenty-three fucking centimeters. A lime is roughly five centimeters; a regular orange with the skin on it is ten centimeters. This was 23 fucking centimeters and surrounded by what felt like some kind of fluid. We were told the mass was "palpable." Remember that word, because when you are getting hit with the kind of news that takes your breath away and makes your heart beat too fast, words matter. They can make or break you. Details matter. Look up "PALPABLE." Google will tell you it means able to be touched or felt, but usually in the form of a tumor **BENIGN**. Yup, you read that right: benign. At that moment, for those days and nights, that was the keyword we were going for: benign. We were not even going to whisper the "C" word. Nope, not happening.

The ER physician told my parents it could be benign, but his concerned look did not support this statement at all. There was nothing else the ER could do; we would have to look elsewhere for answers. We left the hospital, confused and upset by the unknown mystery that lay ahead.

I remember leaving the ER with my mom and going back to my parents' house for a bit. We sat in the living room, discussing what we had just heard. All of us were listening to Google and whatever else we found out on our research binge. That was going to be our sanity for the next couple of days that turned into over two weeks of waiting for a definitive diagnosis. This was the beginning of the end. The last ride before hell froze over, and stress and anxiety were going to become a way of life. Worry was constant, and my soul hurt with fear.

The norm for my mom and me was to talk on the phone every night after work and usually once during work. Now with Luke, it was definite, and each call began with, "What is that blue-eyed baby boy doing now?" My parents live nine miles from me as well, so stopping by on the way home from work was something I did a lot. This ER visit took place on a Saturday. We did not see my mom's General Practitioner (GP), aka Dr. Cool, until 10:00 am the following Monday. What is great about my mom's GP is that they don't make them this way anymore. I called him on his cell that Sunday to tell him about the ER visit the day before. He was always a straight shooter and has a great bedside manner. His words were, "Oh shit," but he held out for hope for the magical word "benign."

The four of us went that Monday morning. I guess I should say five because we had Luke in his stroller. Our doctor made some small talk with us, we had a couple laughs, and then we got to business. He was shocked by how distended my mom's belly was; she looked five months pregnant. I couldn't believe it either. I didn't understand how I hadn't noticed it before, but she had been hiding it with extra-large sweatshirts for months. I had just seen her on Easter at my sister's house, and I had not noticed. None of us noticed. He palpated the mass, did some necessary tests. He had already reviewed the CAT scan results from the ER two days before. I remember him giving the "speech" of, "It's sometimes benign. You need to go to a specialist." But then the final doom came into the room. He referred us to an oncologist, Dr. X, and a surgeon gynecologist/oncologist who I'll call Dr. Z and her partner.

These are two distinct roles. An oncologist treats all types of cancer. The surgeon gynecologist/oncologist treats cancer located in female reproductive organs. We did not want those damn referrals, but this was not a choice. We had lots to do, and we did not have much time to wait. We still thought it might be benign—it had to be benign. Even though our Dr. Cool had told us it could be benign, his face betrayed just how concerned he truly was. Non-verbal communication and eye contact are very important when you are dealing with doctors. Dr. Cool looked at his file many times while he spoke to us. If I were to guess, the ER doctor said he suspected the mass was cancer. Dr. Cool has a couple of modes and when it is a more serious issue, you can tell. He jokes less and looks at his files more, reducing eye contact. Don't get me wrong. He is one of the best doctors I've ever known, and I still use him to this day. But he was more guarded that day. In his heart of hearts, he knew. Just getting these referrals gave us less hope, but your mind plays games with you, and we held onto hope by a thread. Enter the frustration of only being a number in a massive world of other sick people. You are no longer unique.

Our first appointment was with the oncologist/gynecologist, and it was not an easy one to get. I called numerous times, staying on hold for many minutes, as the waiting list was a month long. This wait was the first learning experience I had on this journey. You can't take "no" for an answer. You have to do whatever it takes to be seen, including planting yourself in a doctor's office. You are only one of fifty patients, and your case is not special to them. You are just another victim of this horrible disease called cancer. You have to advocate for your loved one, and waiting can be dangerous, emotionally and physically. Through persistence and a little bit of attitude, we secured an appointment with the oncologist/gynecologist on May 7th.

Again, we went to this appointment as a family: Mom, Dad, my sister, Luke, and myself. Dragging a baby through hospitals was not fun, but he did offer us a good distraction from the hell my mom was going through. We attended many appointments as a family, particularly the big ones and the firsts. We worked together as a cohesive unit throughout my mother's entire illness.

My mom had not been to a gynecologist in forty years. Yes, you read that right: forty years. She had me and never looked back. Let's face it—going to the gynecologist sucks. My mom was old school and saw no need to go even though she had lost friends to female cancer. Who wants to do annual checkups? When she entered the room and saw the famous seat with the stirrups, she immediately got anxious. We tried to make light of it with jokes, but she wasn't feeling our nervous humor. Dr. Z had an exam room and then a discussion office, because unfortunately, in her line of work and specialty, it is common that long, difficult conversations often have to follow an examination. The exam room was hospital white and clean, with some female anatomy models on the counter and the normal sanitary tools used for exams. The smell was of bleach, freshly wiped down from the previous patient. I wondered what news they had gotten?

Dr. Z was of Iranian descent and very reputable. She was, I would guess, in her mid 40s, had a thick Arabic accent, and did not mince words. Even with the accent, her English was very good, so understanding was not a problem While she tried to demonstrate empathy in her demeanor, she was very direct in her message execution. I think part of this was cultural and some was just the specialty she was in. Quite frankly, there is no time for warm and fuzzy with any cancer, and particularly not with ovarian.

Through the beauty of the internet and my obsession with researching anything to do with ovarian cancer, I already knew her legacy before we met her, and it was impressive. She was not only a great physician, but a published researcher looking for a cure and preventative testing for this "silent killer." When we were allowed to go back into the room, Dr. Z was calling it cancer. She did not say she was one hundred percent certain, but looking back, I think she knew and was trying to prepare us for the future. There were too many of us to fit in her office, so we listened in the exam room. I remember the pit in my stomach. The silence in the room as she told us she was pretty confident it was indeed cancer. At this point, I felt it was too early to make that call. I was still betting on benign, still hoping for a miracle, and I was both sad and pissed at what we were being told. We didn't like her for that. I remember saying to my sister, "This woman is the grim reaper. Why is she so fucking negative?" I can admit it today: I didn't care for Dr. Z the first couple months of my mom's battle with this horrible disease. She wasn't telling me what I wanted to hear. Unfortunately, this "grim reaper" was one hundred percent right about every hypothesis she made regarding my mother. Not just the diagnosis, but also the words that she repeatedly echoed: "This is not a friendly cancer." At the time, I thought that was a stupid thing to say. What cancer is friendly? I didn't know it at the time, but Dr. Z turned out to be the best asset to my mom's healthcare team we had, her greatest advocate and a consummate professional.

Some people can go on living normal lives, and there are excellent treatment options, but not so much for ovarian, especially when you are diagnosed late in the game, because the symptoms often show up similar to those for gastroesophageal reflux disease or GERD. Therefore, women ignore them, doctors prescribe antacids and go on until they wind up in the last stages of the disease. In my mom's case, that meant a 23-centimeter pelvic mass and distention like she was five months pregnant.

There were two options: one was to do a biopsy, confirm the carcinoma and treat the cancer with roughly three to four chemotherapy treatments (neoadjuvant chemotherapy) to shrink the mass in preparation for removal at a later date. The second option was to do a lot of preoperative testing and schedule surgery to remove this mass immediately. We wanted to get this out "yesterday." To do that, she needed a lot of pre-op testing.

There is no "immediately" in healthcare. This was another important lesson we learned the hard way—that maintaining your health and taking care of yourself is crucial. We are all guilty of putting physicals and medical tests off.

We all left this appointment feeling nervous and hopeless, and although nobody would admit it, we all knew it was cancer. We decided the best course of action was to get the mass out and proceed with the necessary steps for surgery. The doctor told us we needed to get this tumor out, but first, Mom had to undergo years of avoided testing, including a mammogram, endoscopy, colonoscopy, bone marrow test, endless blood work, a bone density test; you name it, they tested it. Thankfully we got them done in short order.

On May 11th, we returned to our general practitioner for preoperative blood work and to get his sign-off for an EKG, an oxygen level test, and surgery. Our goal was a tentative date of May 17th for surgery. Included in all labs for Mom was a test called CA 125. CA-125 is a biomarker for ovarian cancer that is often elevated in the blood of people with ovarian cancer. It is important to understand that while the CA-125 blood test is useful when diagnosing and monitoring people with ovarian cancer, a CA-125 test alone is not an accurate diagnostic tool. Unfortunately, no single, reliable diagnostic tool exists to detect and diagnose ovarian cancer. My mom's number at this point was 436 with a WNL (within normal limits) range of 0-24, but again, it is a limited diagnostic tool and can't be used alone to diagnose ovarian cancer. You can have a number in the thousands and have a low-grade low stage cancer, and a smaller number and be stage four. Their hope in monitoring it is for the number to go down with any kind of treatment that they throw at you.

On May 12th, Mom had a mammogram and a bone density test. Sixty-eight years old and her first mammogram.

Many don't know this, but female cancers tend to spread to the breasts. I knew a woman who had ovarian cancer and survived it, only to get breast cancer three months after her hair grew back. The mammogram was clean; I can only imagine how mortified my mom was having this test. She was from a generation where this was certainly not the norm. Hey, while we are at it, we know she has bad rheumatoid, so let's see if she has osteoporosis on the same day with a bone density. Yep, as suspected, it was moderate to severe, but she never complained, and remember: she was carrying trays of spaghetti and waiting tables until the day we went to the emergency room.

On May 13th, she had an endoscopy and colonoscopy. The endoscopy revealed she had a very large hiatal hernia, esophagitis, gastritis, and the colonoscopy revealed she had diverticulitis and hemorrhoids, but otherwise, everything was okay. On May 14th, she had a surgical pre-op appointment and a bone marrow test that was very painful. The bone marrow test revealed that her bone marrow couldn't produce enough red blood cells, white blood cells, or platelets. It was a very rare form of acute myeloid leukemia or AML. Who knew? No wonder she was anemic for years, and *always* tired.

But she's never stopped working.

This grueling test schedule indicates how dedicated we were to making the surgery happen as soon as possible. One highlight on all the reports was "there is nothing to compare it to," because she never had any baselines for these previous tests. Given everything they found in pre-op testing, the plan was that they would "try" to repair the hernia during the debulking process, but it was the least of our worries. "Debulking" is the formal word for cleaning out cancer to get "clean" margins, aka, gutting you. She was scheduled for surgery on May

17th. One might ask, why the hell do you have to go through so much testing before surgery? Just get the shit out? Well, at this point, you are no longer in charge of your life because you are fighting for it.

They admitted her on May 16th, the night before, and surgery was scheduled for the morning of the 17th. Unfortunately, her pre-op blood showed platelet chemistry of 1.2 million, and your WNL (within normal limits) for adult platelets is between 150,000 and 450,000 per microliter of blood. Hers was a condition called thrombocytosis.

Thrombocytosis during surgery can be a death sentence, as too many platelets in the blood puts you at high risk for a heart attack or stroke via blood clot. Because of this condition, my mom was extremely weak, and the medical team called the surgery off because of the risks. To say we were disappointed is an understatement. This would be strike one of one many.

On May 19th, they ordered a temporary plasmapheresis catheter placement. This procedure is done in interventional radiology. It is not easy; they put a catheter in your jugular vein for many kinds of treatments. My mom was fully awake with only some numbing agents. On this day, she also had a CT angiography with and without contrast. The results showed no evidence of pulmonary embolism, the hiatal hernia was filled with a lot of ascites, and there was some evidence of fluid in the lungs and liver abnormalities. At this time, they did nothing with these results. They felt they were "reactive" to cancer, and the hernia was the least of our worries.

The last procedure on this very long day was platelet apheresis. What the hell is platelet apheresis? It is a big machine similar to dialysis, wherein your blood is drawn from your body into this sterile machine, the platelets are removed, and the remaining blood components are then returned to your body. It is kind of like a rinse cycle, but instead of cleaning clothes, it removes extra junk that can kill you. This was supposed to be done on an outpatient basis, but it took all day, and by about seven pm, my mom was wiped out. The tech called the hospitalist, and there were "no rooms" for admission, so we would have to go through the Emergency Room. That wasn't happening, because she was already in a weakened state, and going through the Emergency Room with everyone sick was an invitation to get a cold, flu, or any other type of infection. Thankfully, this tech/nurse had a heart of gold, called in a favor, and found us a room to be admitted, so we did not have to go through the Emergency Room. Always be kind to your nurses and techs. Be nice to everyone, but especially your nurses. They can make or break you; they are the cohesive tissue and glue between the patient and the doctor. They are the captains of the team, hands down.

Surgery was scheduled for the next morning, May 20th. D-day was finally here, but perhaps it wasn't. We (my dad, my sister, and myself) arrived at her room early in the morning as she was the six am case, and we found an exasperated, anxious, and emotionally drained Mom. The surgeons made the decision again that surgery was too risky and that my mom was too weak. At this moment, there were no doctors in the room, and I immediately saw red. This is the norm for me. I wanted to know who made the choice to fucking cancel surgery, why, and where the fuck this person was. My dad was equally annoyed, but he was not as loud as I was, and my sister was annoyed but handled it, I'd say, the best out of all of us.

You will see my reactive theme throughout this book and I won't apologize for it. Sometimes it is necessary to get shit done. My dad even had his lucky "Get 'er Done" hat on. About an hour went by, and my mom probably told me two or three times to relax, and finally my mom's team of doctors came in—the lead oncologist, the two gynecology/oncology surgeons, and their "band" of students, who, I have to be honest, were getting annoying. While I understand that you have to learn somewhere and it was a teaching hospital, having strangers (medical students) gawk at you while you're crying, having the life sucked out of you, hearing the shittiest news ever, and being told of your unknown prognosis wasn't very fun, nor did it need an audience. You are just a number: a file number, a case. You are what they hope they never have to go through. You're an example of why preventative care matters; you are just another case study, a learning opportunity, and probably an upcoming research project or exam.

I digress. The file notes: "Based on her progressive symptoms, the extent of the disease in the imaging studies and the tumor board decided neoadjuvant therapy would be more appropriate at the present time. A 68-year-old woman with ADVANCED PROBABLE OVARIAN CANCER WITH HEMATOLOGIC abnormalities, which appear to be reactive in nature" needs to fucking wait. "Due to her advanced disease and poor performance status, the patient will remain in the hospital and will be receiving neoadjuvant systemic chemotherapy with Carboplatin and Taxol."

Strike fucking two.

Plan B was neoadjuvant chemotherapy, if and when they received a positive biopsy. The "plan" was to do three to six cycles of neoadjuvant therapy. Three to fucking six cycles. Oh, and P.S, it will be easy, they said. We were told usually you don't feel any "illness" from the chemo until after the third or fourth round. Remember that. Although the doctors gave this process high success rates, our hope was dwindling fast. The next step was a tumor biopsy. This is where the real "fun" began. Dr. Z put in the order for the biopsy around ten am on May 20th, the day the surgery was canceled. They also sent her to interventional radiology for paracentesis for therapeutic purposes and comfort. What the heck is paracentesis? It is the process of removing ascitic fluid **for** diagnostic or therapeutic purposes. They use a fairly large needle or catheter. It is not really a comfortable procedure even though they use a numbing agent on the skin. But the relief the patient feels after getting all of that fluid out of them is a necessary and rewarding evil. Remember, the ascites surrounded the tumor, and on any given day because of the aggressiveness of the disease, she was carrying the 23 cm tumor and roughly a gallon of fluid on top of it, which made moving, breathing, and eating difficult. This fluid built up and made her feel full all the time, all while she continued to lose weight.

During the night she had an irregular EKG, so she also had a cardiac consult. "Patient was not a smoker, drinker, or on any exercise regime. She was working until three weeks ago when she became very uncomfortable due to her increased abdominal size." Two electrocardiograms on May 20th showed sinus tachycardia. The CAT scan results did not show anything crazy, but they did put her on a beta- blocker to manage her heart rate. Generally, my mom's vitals were good, and she did not have hypertension. She had hypotension, which means low blood pressure. It generally was not problematic unless she got out of bed quickly; she might feel a little dizzy, but this was never a concern for any doctor.

On May 21ˢᵗ, Mom had a nephrology consult with a kidney doctor due to her high platelet count. Her blood also showed high WBC (white blood cells), low iron, and anemia. Anemia and cancer generally walk hand-in-hand. On May 22nd, she was very anemic and required her first blood transfusion. I'll never forget the first time they mentioned that she might need blood; she was concerned about how much it cost. She was always worried about bills and how much all of this care was costing. I remember telling her she could have my blood and not to worry about it. Thankfully, my parents had pretty good insurance.

On May 24ᵗʰ, again, she had paracentesis, and this time they also did cytology on the fluid they removed. Cytology is the exam of a single cell type, as often found in fluid specimens. You know the biopsy that was ordered the morning of the 20th? Keep in mind at this time, we still did not have a final diagnosis. Doctor Z's cancer diagnosis was based on all clinical evidence in pictures, labs, CAT scans, and presentation of symptoms, but we had no biopsy from pathology. Dr. Z ordered the biopsy when she left my mom's room the morning the second scheduled surgery was canceled. Four fucking days ago with a 24-hour turnaround. While a couple of days may not sound like not a big deal, when you are going through this and trying to keep a positive outlook even though each turn keeps kicking you in the teeth, an hour feels like a year. They tested the ascites for carcinogens, and it came back positive for "adenocarcinoma with mucin secreting cells." We were never told "officially." We were still running on hypotheses and physical evidence, blood work, signs, and some common effects that my mom demonstrated that indicated cancer, but we still had no diagnosis. Interventional radiology was given orders to place a PICC line in her at this time for future chemotherapy.

While I'd like to say we knew what was coming, we were clueless. All of the internet research, late-night chat rooms, and telling ourselves the doctors were wrong and this was going to be benign— none of it could prepare us for the poor nurse who drew the short straw and entered my mom's room on May 25th. She entered pulling an IV with a yellow substance hanging in the bag and she was dressed up like she was going into chemical warfare. What the fuck? If you are not sitting, you might want to pull up a chair now. The nurse came in, and we had seen her before, a lovely woman in a chemical warfare suit telling my mom, and I quote, "Okay, Ms. Burns, we have your chemotherapy, and we are going to start now." Wait, what? Back the hell up. Chemotherapy? We knew it was a possibility, but we never had a diagnosis. We never heard from the doctors, never had a stage, prognosis, type? Are you fucking kidding me now? My sister said to the nurse, "Why are you dressed like that?"

"Because this is poison, and I can't get it on me. Ms. Burns, are you ready to begin?"

What? Now, mind you, it was not the nurse's fault. She was just following the chart, following the doctor's orders, but where was the doctor telling the patient the diagnosis? What stage of this horrible C-word did she have? What was her prognosis? How bad was it? How long was this chemotherapy going to take? What in the actual fuck? So, I immediately got on the phone, calling my mom's oncologist, Dr X. I left a not-so-nice message with his practice and expected him to show up before he left for the day and explain what the biopsy showed. We waited five days, not 24 hours, and this was how we found out? A poor nurse doing her job who can't answer clinical questions but can only tell you what she is putting into your mother's body is fucking poison? This was another case of poor communication and follow up, and a good example of how you're only a number. This was unbelievable to me; this lack of empathy and explanation from a professional was unacceptable.

What if she had been alone? What about the many patients who are alone when they get news like that? What happens to them? You will see in the rest of this book many other examples of poor or wrong communication. While I understand the job of an oncologist is probably one of the hardest in medicine because they are up against an enemy that changes in each case and are often blamed when treatments do not work, this was basic patient-doctor relationship stuff. It was communication 101, the very keystone to patient trust.

After the initial diagnosis of ovarian cancer, Stage 3C, Mom immediately became pretty depressed. She tried to keep a stiff upper lip and was in the game to win, but it was a hard pill to swallow and there were a lot of unknowns. In Stage 3C ovarian cancer, the cancer is found in one or both ovaries, as well as in the abdomen's lining, or it has spread to lymph nodes in the abdomen. We all tried everything to cheer her up with positive reinforcement, telling her, "You can beat this," sharing statistics, bringing the grandchildren to visit, citing what we learned on our internet research— you name it, we tried it.

This was her first admission of many. It included a lot of confusion, stress, changed plans, medical procedures, and testing, and then she finally received an "official" diagnosis and treatment options. She got her first round of chemotherapy before she was discharged on May 26th.

When my sister picked Mom up after that first round of inpatient chemotherapy, she was doing well; she was dressed, had her hair done, makeup on, and I thought, *Okay, maybe we can do this*. What I didn't know then was that it's usually rounds two and three of chemotherapy that hit you the worst. They treated her with a "normal" chemo regimen for ovarian cancer, but years later, when I went to the genetic counselor to inquire about her case and plan for my own hysterectomy, I found out that she didn't have normal ovarian cancer. She had sarcomas, very rare and very deadly sarcomas, and the shit they were treating her with never would have touched them. Unfortunately, when they went to aspirate the tumor for biopsy, they got a sample from the ascites and did not get a sample from the tumor. Therefore, they designed the chemotherapy based on the ascites, not the fucking tumor. This turned out to be a huge mistake.

THINGS WE LEARNED IN MAY:

1. Keep in close contact with the treatment team. Keep a log of names, specialties, areas of expertise, what condition they are treating, floors they work on, phone numbers.

2. Get to know the nurses on the floor. They are so important to the process if your loved one is critically ill. Nurses, in my experience, can be more important than the doctors. Get to know them, treat them well, ask questions, and get names.

3. Ask a lot of questions and write down the answers. Your loved one does not have the mental capacity to remember everything and answer all the questions thrown at them when they are going through a medical crisis like this. They might not hear everything the doctors say. The stress of the diagnosis impacts their ability to listen and sort out what is important, and they become really confused. They also don't want to hear this news about their fate. Medical terminology is often difficult to understand. That is why it is critical to always ask and if necessary, ask again and get it into a language that everyone understands.

4. Do not allow four days to get test results for a biopsy when cancer is a possibility. Time is everything. You have to keep following up even if it means going down to where the test took place. In this process, you may "annoy" people but what is the alternative? Try your best to be patient, but remember you are not there to make friends. It

can be a matter of life and death.

5. Write down and keep track of ALL medications prescribed, including IV. Write down the dosage, frequency, PRN prescription (pro re nata), whether it is scheduled or as needed, which medication is for what patient need, any special instructions, etc. When discharged, do not leave the hospital without all your necessary prescriptions in hand. Do not rely on the nurse or doctor to call them in to the pharmacy. If your loved one was prescribed pain medication, each state has different rules about prescribing with the opioid crisis. It is very important to someone suffering to confirm the script is where you plan to pick it up before you leave the hospital. Make sure you keep this medication log with you at all times, and include any allergies or side effects from medications that you have experienced.

6. Spend as much time at the hospital as you can, especially in the beginning of an ordeal like ours. This is important for many reasons. First, you need to support your family member, as any hospital stay can be a frightening experience. Second, you need to ensure the hospital staff knows you are NOT a family that is going to go away and trust the system. Successful treatment and reducing errors require everyone working together as a team to ensure everyone is on the same page.

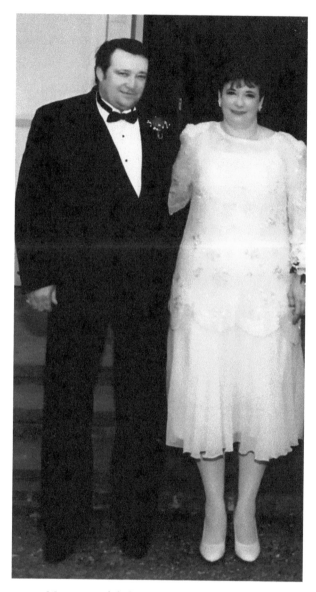

My mom and dad at my sister's wedding, 1990.

3

JUNE

Chemotherapy is one of the only known treatments for cancer in the western world. Don't get me wrong; there are pills, radiation, and some holistic options, but the treatment of choice for cancer is chemotherapy. It boggles my mind how behind we are in this. Chemo works by attacking cancerous cells, but unfortunately, it also attacks the healthy cells, making the patient weak. The side effects vary; some people take it very well and go on with life as though nothing has changed, while others suffer as my mother did. She got her first round in the hospital, and that was "easy."

On June 2nd, before getting her second treatment, Mom had to go to interventional radiology to get a PICC line change. This was scheduled to be done via outpatient, but while she was there, she became uncomfortable, so they also ordered paracentesis. Ascites can make the patient lose weight, nutrients, albumin, have problems breathing, swallowing, experience weakness, etc. The first time they did this in interventional radiology in May, they took about seven liters out of my mother. Seven liters is the equivalent of 1.8 gallons. The substance looks like beer with a "head," if you can believe it. Unfortunately, it's a common side effect of cancer, and as the cancer progresses, paracentesis becomes more and more necessary for the patient's comfort, ability to breathe easily, and eat. In theory, the chemotherapy should begin to "dry" up the development of this nasty fluid buildup if it is effective.

At one point, Mom was having it done about two to three times a week. This time, after this process was over, my sister noticed Mom's breathing was a bit labored, so when I got lucky and happened to catch my mom's oncologist, Dr. X in the hallway, I asked him to come to interventional radiology to look at her. He thought she was fine but decided to admit her to cardiology for a review and ultrasounds the next day, to rule out DVTs (deep vein thrombosis) or pulmonary embolisms. These are the unpleasant complications that coexist with cancer. Now, keep in mind, it was not a doctor who diagnosed this; it was my sister who noticed the labored breathing and insisted she be seen.

When we got Mom up to cardiology, we went through the usual patient bill of rights, HIPAA forms, etc. A young resident (again, this was a teaching hospital) came in to sit with my mother and go over her patient health care proxy. He had another student with him. He asked Mom, "If something happens while you are on this floor, do you want us to take any lifesaving actions?" Mom, who was on Ativan and pain meds at the time, answered, "Do nothing if there is no hope."

What the hell did that mean?

The student marked his folder and left. The entire process took less than five minutes. I asked Mom, "Do you know what you just told him? You told him if you have a cardiac arrest in the middle of the night, not to do anything."

"No, I did not," Mom said.

What my mom meant was that she did not want a ventilator or a stomach tube if she was brain dead. That was in her health care proxy for years. I walked to the nursing station and made the resident come back to Mom's room to explain her wishes more clearly. He updated her chart and was told to take any lifesaving measures if, God forbid, she needed them. What if I had not been there?

You have to be careful at teaching hospitals because people are continually coming in and out, looking at the patient for five minutes, and then you end up with a bill for $500 and way too many chefs in the kitchen who really do not know your loved one's case. While I understand that this is necessary for learning, it is my experience that you have to be very alert and mindful of all of your interactions. Later, I would look at the medical bills from my mother's various hospital stays and see shitloads of names I didn't recognize who did absolutely nothing for her but be in the room. The patient also becomes part of the teaching process. You know this if you have ever watched *Grey's Anatomy*: you, as the patient are like a sick fish in a fishbowl, with many fishermen questioning you, hoping to impress the doctor on call with an answer to win the prize, but the fish just floats, feeling sicker and growing tired, gasping for air and answers. It can be very unsettling.

It gets better. As I was leaving, I don't know why I did it, but I looked at her identification bracelet. You should know that everything depends on that bracelet/patient ID. The bracelet has a barcode that serves as your medical record, including medications, labs, allergies, history, insurance, and demographics. Instead of Constance E. Burns, there was another woman's name on the bracelet. I should have taken a picture, but instead, I got the head nurse. As soon as they heard, they came in and cut the bracelet off very quickly. Again, what if we had not been there? Would she have been sent down for an angiogram in the middle of the night or another cardiac procedure? Could she have been given meds that would have killed her because they were treating the wrong patient? I did report it, but the patient advocate didn't want to hear it from me. There's one patient advocate for the entire hospital, and of course, that person is biased because the hospital cuts their paycheck.

We finally left after she settled in and waited for them to ultrasound her lungs and legs the next day, looking for blood clots. Surprise, she had bilateral pulmonary embolisms (PE) in each lung and DVTs (deep vein thrombosis) in each leg. My sister called me at work with the results. Mom was very anemic and needed multiple blood transfusions during this hospital stay. The treatment for PEs and DVTs was a daily shot of Lovenox in the stomach. Lovenox is an anticoagulant (blood thinner).

She was discharged from cardiology two days later on June 5th, and she was feeling pretty okay. On June 9th, she went for her daily Lovenox shot, pre-chemo blood work, and scheduled paracentesis. To the tech's surprise, there were no ascites to remove. This was great news. This should indicate that the chemo was starting to really work.

The medical team told us the fluid would probably not stop building around the tumor until well after the second round of chemo, so having this result only after the first was very encouraging. On the same visit, my mom's blood work showed her red blood count up and platelets finally just outside the normal range.

This was the direction we were trying to go. Her white blood cells continued to be high but not astronomical. This was a given due to the cancer and the Neulasta shot. Finally, they told her if she continued to be able to eat and need less frequent paracentesis, they could possibly move her to the pill Coumadin to use as an anticoagulant, so she wouldn't need to go to the hospital every day for the shot. June 9th was a good day, even though just seven days prior, she had been admitted for bilateral pulmonary embolisms and DVTs (deep vein thrombosis) in her legs. This is just one example of the mental cliff we were hanging on. As I said before, every negative hypothesis or worry her oncologist/gynecologist Dr. Z. had had come true. If there were a book on all the bad complications that can coexist with the diagnosis of ovarian cancer, my poor mom would eventually experience every one. It seemed that with every step she might have taken forward on any given day, for some reason, the lousy cancer would rear its ugly head and set her another step back. I guess what I'm trying to say is any "celebrations" we had from this point on would be countered with a swift kick to the teeth.

We were now getting ready for the second round of outpatient chemotherapy, scheduled for June 15th. Welcome to the chemo suite. "Suite" is a funny word. It makes you think high end, fancy, a wet bar, butler service, room service, luxury tub, linens, the works. Not so much. We proceeded to the chemo "suite" for Mom's first outpatient chemo. The nurses in the suite are wonderful, some of the most caring, knowledgeable, compassionate folks you will ever meet. You generally share a room with someone like you who is fighting a battle. Cancer is an equal opportunity disease, and you see all walks of life in the suite. For the most part, people are pretty sick. Some can be your age and others much younger. The treatment would last six long hours. Benadryl was given first to open the veins and prevent any allergic reaction. Chemotherapy was six bags. I remember bringing Luke to this treatment in the last hour, and he was really good at making people, including my mother, smile.

At this point, my mom's hair started falling out in clumps on her pillow, and my sister shaved her head. Insurance would have paid for wigs, but she didn't want to wear one. To this day, I don't know how my sister did it. This is what I meant—that during times like these, we balanced each other with strengths and weaknesses. I really don't think I could have shaved her head. Not only because I would have completely messed it up, but, more importantly, I knew I could not emotionally handle it. No fucking way. During this stage, we all had hope as a family unit. We found out later that it was misguided, but we all had faith that this ugly mass was indeed shrinking, that the chemo was working, and we would soon be able to have the surgery to remove it. We were preparing for this day in every way. Mentally, physically, we even forced my poor mom onto the treadmill. Why, you ask? Because we were trying to keep my mom mentally and physically healthy. Looking back, the second treatment really had a negative effect on my mom. It was at this time, I think, that she mentally gave up.

I remember one particular phone conversation with my mom where she was really down. She seemed defeated, felt like shit, said she looked like shit and didn't have high hopes for any future. You could cut the tension with a knife because her voice was low and she was holding back crying, and I was doing the same, except it was my job to stay strong and positive. I chose to give her some tough love. I remember saying things like, "Are you ready to die? Are you just going to give up like that?" I was trying to hit her with guilt when what I really should have been doing was listening. I thought if I went down the negative road with her, I would not be helping her fight, and we needed her to fight. We were not throwing in the towel any time soon, and if I had to be the bad guy, then I'd be the bad guy. At the same time, I tried to encourage her with the fact that we had "just started the fight and everything that I read on the internet gave her a good chance at winning this war."

To this day I still feel bad about this approach. But I felt as though I had no choice. I was desperate. I also tried forcing her to eat, trying to shove alternative medicines on her—green drinks, organic mushrooms that smelled like dirt, you name it— but the lousy cancer had its hooks in and was not letting up.

Every day, Mom had to get a Lovenox shot at the hospital at 8:45 am. She was not a morning person (remember, her job was working nights as a waitress, so most mornings she was recovering from the work she'd done until the late hours the night before), but they could not get the Lovenox at home as it was very expensive. It was free if she was injected at the hospital. So, every day she had to go to the hospital for this shot. My sister tried to plan other doctor appointments around it, labs, treatments and paracentesis.

From day one, my sister was sending emails routinely to many friends and family, giving updates on where we were, how Mom was doing, and trying to keep them light and positive. My mom was loved by so many, and the list only grew as time went by. As I look back and read those letters, I am amazed at how my sister captured what was happening on this roller coaster ride from hell.

THINGS WE LEARNED IN JUNE:

1.   Trust, but holy shit, verify. Look what happened that night in cardiology. The student got her health care proxy wrong. Dead wrong. The resident heard what a very depressed and sick patient said and didn't probe to ensure he understood. Little things aren't so little. Humans make mistakes. Nobody is perfect. There is a reason why surgeons will mark the body part you are being operated on before surgery. We have all heard the stories of someone getting the wrong knee replaced. There are a million ways that wrong identity could have gone sideways for my mom. Ten years later, I have probably had ten procedures or major surgeries and hospital admissions. They ask you every day, before any medication, before any procedure and when any new staff comes in, for you to identify yourself, and at that time, they check your bracelet. Make sure this is done. Every time.

2.   Trust your instincts. My sister thought my mom's breathing was labored. I happened to get lucky and see her oncologist in the hallway, and guess what. She had four clots. She was a walking time bomb. Cancer causes clots; it is a known side effect of the disease. Trust your gut, and do not take no for an answer, even if the professional feels that you are possibly overreacting or wrong.

3.   I can't stress this enough: know who is on the medical team. Write everything down. Continue to build your knowledge, especially if your admission is unplanned. This month, my mom was admitted

to cardiology. This was an entirely new group of people. Find out who is responsible for your loved one's care while they are on this floor. How many other patients does that RN have? Does it feel like they are understaffed? What is the patient-nurse ratio? What time do the doctors in charge of your loved one's care usually make rounds? They are usually in the morning, but I can tell you that it can vary significantly in a teaching hospital. I know you are probably thinking, *How the heck am I going to get all that information?* But trust me. It is there if you ask for it. You can't have too much information.

4. You can refuse to be treated by students. It is your right. Advise the team, and put a note on the door. I will tell you that after this resident misinterpreted my mom's medical management, we refused to let any more medical students see my mom. Sorry! We gave it the team try, but you blew it.

4

JULY

This is a direct quote from my sister's July 7th email blast to our friends and family concerning my mom. "Falling down the medical rabbit hole, standing on a carpet and having it ripped out from under you, getting tapped on the shoulder by Divine Intervention and feeling like you were hit on the head by a two-by-four...all of those things sum up this roller coaster ride. But I continue to hope for the light at the end of this tunnel." My sister was once again able to keep a steady hand while my head was exploding.

It was evident that my mom was beginning to really suffer and seemed to be getting worse and not better, both physically and mentally. She was in a lot of physical pain, having difficulty walking and breathing. She was sleeping at all hours and had a significant loss of appetite, nausea, and depression. She was scheduled for the third round of chemotherapy on July 6th, but before the third treatment, we asked for a CAT scan. It was clear we needed to pump the brakes and do some checking. On July 2nd, she got a CAT scan of her chest, pelvis, and abdomen with contrast. The CAT scan was scheduled for 8:30 am, which my mom was not thrilled about, and she had to drink that nasty barium stuff again. They also ordered placement of an inferior vena cava (IVC) into her artery under IV sedation. The simple explanation is that it's a mesh-like material that looks like an umbrella, and it's used to catch blood clots for those prone to them or with heart disease. They also gave her steroids to combat the exhaustion that comes with chemo. Remember, at this point, she had two rounds of chemo behind her. Still, we saw her becoming sicker and weaker each passing day, so we wanted to see if the neoadjuvant chemo treatment had had any impact on this lousy tumor. If the answer was no, we needed to change the course, not put her through anymore chemotherapy, and look for alternatives.

On July 6th, my sister and my mom went to the oncologist office to get pre-chemo labs and saw the nurse practitioner. Dr. X was unavailable, so the nurse practitioner gave my family the CAT scan results that said the tumor had shrunk in half, so we should proceed with the third round of chemo. We were doing a fucking jig. For those hours, for those moments, we felt we could actually breathe a little better. Finally, we saw some light at the end of the tunnel. We were thrilled; soon, she would have the surgery. The mass was now roughly twelve centimeters, and the "debulking" would be a much easier task.

On July 7th, we had an appointment with my mom's surgeon gynecologist/oncologist, Dr. Z, and her partner. Dr. Z told us that the nurse practitioner from the oncologist's office had given us the wrong information. She proceeded to tell us that the mass had not shrunk significantly. Wait, what? Time out. But my mom had the third round of chemo yesterday? We were given the green light and following orders. We were celebrating and actually felt that even though we saw the physical toll it was taking, something was finally working. What the fuck had they missed?

The surgeon compared the first scan from May 1st to the scan on July 2nd, and there was no fucking change. One step forward, two steps back, with a bonus kick to the fucking teeth. Read this again if necessary. This is not a small mistake. We added more poison to an already very ill woman. The entire purpose of the CAT scan was to get some answers to make important treatment choices to reduce suffering. Wasting syndrome was in overdrive, and her poor body and spirit were in rapid decline. Cachexia, also called cancer cachexia or cancer anorexia, is a wasting syndrome. It is the loss of fat and muscle due to a chronic disease, such as cancer, and not eating enough nutrients (malnourishment). Cachexia causes weight loss, loss of appetite, weakness, and fatigue. Remember how I told you to keep track of your loved one's weight? This is one reason why. The lousy cancer takes everything from you, and if the disease does not, the treatment will.

Every day that passed, every hour, Mom was getting weaker, thinner, and sicker. Any hope that she had was gone, and she was tired. We all were tired, but she was visibly disappearing, body and soul, before our eyes. My mom had a decision to make, and we were going to support her no matter what. She opted for the surgery, but we had to wait for the chemo to leave her body; you can't have surgery when your body is filled with poison. So, we would need to wait a month before we could even consider surgery. A month is a long time when you're wasting away. When you get to the point where chemo is making you so exhausted you need steroid shots, your body ends up running on steroids. After this treatment and news, my mom slept most of the day. The goal of this type of treatment was to reduce the tumor size to make the surgery easier, but in reality, all it did was poison a sick woman. I'd call this strike three, and we were into overtime in this terrible game.

There were three scenarios for the surgery's outcome. In the best-case scenario, they would go in, remove most cancer cells and tumors safely, and then administer "clean up" chemo to get any straggler cells. This was the top goal of surgery and what they would call "optimally debulked." The surgery should have resulted in no residual tumors individually measuring more than two centimeters in size.

The second scenario was to go in and take out as much as possible to give Mom better quality of life and relieve the pressure on all her organs, then do more chemo.

The third and worst-case scenario was to go in, find the cancer was too advanced and other vital organs were involved, close her up without taking out the tumor, and attempt to handle it palliatively.

"Palliative care" is not the phrase you want to hear. It is specialized medical care that focuses on providing patients relief from pain and other symptoms of a severe illness, no matter the diagnosis or stage of the disease. Palliative care teams aim to improve the quality of life for both patients and their families. This form of care is offered alongside curative or other treatments you may be receiving. The short definition is that they will do everything possible to keep you comfortable because there is a very high probability that you are not treatable medically. The next step will probably be hospice care and death.

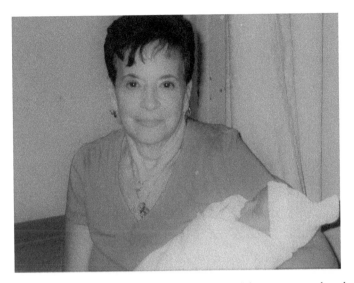

My mom was at my son Luke's birth and 1st birthday party even though she was very sick. He only got 15 months with her.

July 8th is my son Luke's birthday. There was no way my mom was going to miss it. On the following Sunday, the 11th, we had a very small birthday party for him, just immediate family—Anthony's dad, his brother, my niece and nephews, my sister, her husband, and my parents. My sister made a Spiderman cake for Luke. I remember it perfectly. How she still managed to do crafty stuff in this tense, anxiety-ridden environment in which we were all living still boggles my mind. I guess she was stronger because she had to be. My nephews (her children) were 8 and 12, and my mom meant the world to them; so she kept the severity of my mom's illness from them as long as she could. As far as they knew, my mom had something wrong with her stomach and eventually needed surgery. I don't know when she told them it was cancer, but I would bet it was close to this time. They're smart kids, and my mom had no hair.

We all were just trying to act as normal as possible, but in reality, we were all dying inside with my mother. It was July in New York so it was a hot day; my mom came and struggled to walk up the driveway, and my dad held her arm. Unlike her usual social self, she beelined straight into our house, sat inside in the living room, and did not go outside to see anyone on the patio. While we are definitely not the *big entrance everyone gets a hug* type, it was not like my mom to avoid everyone. It was kind of like she saw Luke and then was ready to go home. She didn't feel good. She was tired, nauseated, and depressed. I knew she forced herself to come. She was only there about fifteen minutes and struggling to keep her eyes open in the chair when I told her to go into my bedroom and rest. She did. She didn't interact with anyone, just slept, and she and my dad left within a couple hours. Everyone outside tried to keep a stiff upper lip and not make a big deal about it. Again, all of us were putting up a front to celebrate my son with pits in our stomachs. This behavior was not my mom at all. She was weak, tired, suffering, and emotionally shot. For the remaining days in July, waiting for surgery after hearing probably the worst news possible, my mom fell into a dark depression. She was down to 129 pounds, filled with a lot of fluid and a huge, ugly mass that had not fucking shrunk like we were told it would.

On July 26th, we had an appointment with my mom's surgical gynecologist/oncologist, Dr. Z. She and her team were having a hard time getting all of the medical specialties she needed in the operating room to do my mom's surgery. There was a risk of bowel perforation, so she required a colon surgeon; she had a large hiatal hernia, so she needed a gastrointestinal surgeon, even though that was the least of our worries. They wanted to try to fix it when they had her open. They needed both oncologist/gynecologist surgeons, nurses, and an anesthesiologist.

It was July 26th, and we had been waiting since May 1st, following their suggested treatment plan, and it was not working. The surgery would be scheduled and then canceled; they told us we might be looking at the fall. The fall? Were they looking at this woman? It was the end of fucking July! How many fucking times can you get kicked in the face? We were all in Dr. Z's office, and my mom was defeated, not only by cancer, but now also by administrative bullshit. I wasn't taking fall as an answer. By now, I was a maniac. This surgery could not wait.

As my family sat in Dr. Z's office I got up. I snapped, and everyone around me knew it. All of the surgeons and schedulers sat in an office at the end of the hall. I opened the door, took a chair from the waiting room, and parked myself in the scheduling office that had about ten administrative assistants in it, and said I wasn't leaving until they scheduled the surgery. A couple of the staff told me that I had to leave and that it was not an area that I could be in, but I told them I would fucking sleep there if I had to and to feel free to call security. The look on my face was indignant rage. They were now telling me October. Are you fucking kidding me? Every day she was dying. I would have slept there, I would have been carried out by security, I didn't fucking care.

The doctor knew we were at the end of our rope; Mom was crying, Dad was pissed off, my sister tried to be the peacekeeper and help keep everyone's emotions in check in the examination room. At this point, Dr. Z pulled out her cell phone and stated pacing up and down the hall making phone calls. She had my family in her examination room and me in the scheduling room, and she was in the middle, trying to get my mom scheduled because she knew that time was not on our side, and I was probably one step away from getting myself in trouble.

My poor mom was defeated. She told us we would not leave the hospital without a date, and by the end of our visit, we had one. August 4th. We were so grateful. Sometimes it takes a village, but you can't give up or take no for an answer. You also must remember that when it comes to life and death, you are not there to make friends. The administrators were very mad that I was in their space making demands and that I infiltrated their "process," but at that point, I didn't give a single fuck.

Even though Mom had an appointment for the surgery, her albumin was very low, and her weight continued to drop. Albumin is a blood protein that is very important to plasma. Low albumin can be caused by many things; in my mom's case, it was malabsorption, malnutrition, and malignancy, aka fucking cancer. We tried to get her to consume protein, green drinks, and Boost, but she could not put on weight. Her surgeon was very concerned about these counts, so she admitted Mom into the hospital for total parenteral nutrition (TPN). This is intravenous nutrition. She did this for a week before the surgery. During this time, her mood was okay. She was scared, but in slightly better spirits than she had been. The TPN was given to her around the clock and they kept doing blood work.

From the start of this walk-through hell, my sister and I were in constant communication. She watched my son and took care of my mom and dad during the day while I was at work. I would generally go to the hospital in the evening and spend time with my mom. Mom was more worried about me, telling me to go home and spend time with my son. "You worked all day, get some rest," etc. Many times, she had to kick me out and I got home around nine or ten pm. As I said in my letter to my mother, this was a time when I was running on empty, gutted, helpless and hopeless.

Little did I know that my anxiety and sleepless nights were only going to get worse. I visited her at the hospital at various times, depending on the day. Thankfully, due to a very understanding employer, I was able to come and go as I needed to. We were regulars on the 11th floor and knew many of the nurses. They saw a concerned, tight family that was there every day, and even though it is the very fucking last place you want to visit, somehow, we were there so much. It was welcoming because of the nurses. The floor is made up of critically ill patients waiting to die, and others that are pulling bags of chemo around like it's saline and are ready to get discharged. During one admission, my mom was not in a private room and her roommate had oral cancer. She could not speak and was blind. I never saw any visitors. It was absolutely heartbreaking. I would sometimes go in to her space and say hello and try to perk her up because she could hear, but it was beyond tragic. Nobody deserves to die alone.

For a while she was doing better and lots of people were coming to visit, but around Saturday, that changed. Her abdomen began filling with that ugly ascites again, making walking a chore and breathing more labored. We were concerned, the surgeons more so.

THINGS WE LEARNED IN JULY:

1.   If your loved one has to go to chemo, bring something they can munch on or some magazines. If they have a hobby like crochet, bring it, or even a deck of cards. You can also ask for anti-anxiety or sleeping meds if it's going to take a long time.

2.   Check and double-check the diagnosis. We were given inaccurate information about Mom's tumor shrinking; this gave us false hope. Had we known the truth, we would not have put Mom through another round of chemo that wasn't having any positive impact on her cancer.

3.   If your loved one is very sick, you're going to spend a lot of time at the hospital. Try to have patience with the nurses and staff. This may not always be easy, as mistakes do happen, but you will learn quickly that nothing happens without a cooperative nurse. Try to befriend a couple of good nurses. I can't say it enough. They are so important to the care of your loved one, and good ones can help you navigate the maze in the hospital. We had a very special friendship with one nurse in oncology/gynecology—I'll call her Flower. Flower kept us in the "know," and she was an advocate and cheerleader for my mom and my family. She visited my mom after her shift just to sit with her, talk, and be there for her when the family had to leave after visiting hours. You don't find too many people like Flower, and I will never be able to thank her enough. She also stuck her neck out for us

when it may have caused herself problems with her employer. I hope this book will find her, and even though I have kept her name private, she will know it is her and that we are forever grateful to her.

4. Make sure that the medical team knows about nutrition intake. The meals are delivered to the patient's room and picked up by kitchen services, but they are not checked to see whether the patient has eaten or not. It was very common that my mom would return full trays of food and only ingest maybe half of a Boost. It is important to let the medical team know these things. If you are with your loved one all day in the hospital, keep open communication with everyone, even if it is one-way. If you noticed that they had breakthrough pain (the patient feels pain even though they are medicated) let the medical staff know; if you saw breakthrough nausea (the patient is nauseated even though they have been treated for nausea) let them know; if they had difficulty ambulating to the bathroom, inform them. Unfortunately, nurses do rounds roughly once an hour if you're lucky, and a lot goes unnoticed and unchecked. I don't blame the nurses; I blame the system.

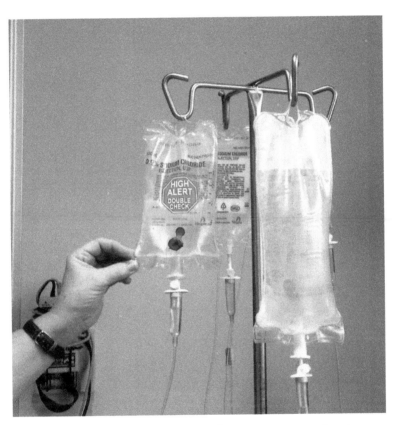

Chemotherapy is poison. Sometimes the treatment is worse than the disease.

5

AUGUST

On August 4th, we finally got around to the surgery. Mom was in the hospital for nine days before the surgery, getting much needed nutrition.

Debulking is a common term for the removal of all or most bulky cancerous tumors. In the case of ovarian cancer, this is usually the goal, and unfortunately, it often has to be repeated depending on the diagnosis. On the evening of August 3rd, around 9:30 p.m. Dr. Z. came in and asked me to speak to her in the hall. This could not be good. She told me that Mom was very sick, and she was not comfortable with her case. She said tomorrow we needed to be in the operating room by six a.m., and the operation would probably be palliative. Palliative? What? Just for comfort, not a cure? Short term? What was the fucking point then? What kind of bullshit was this, and being told just a few hours before? I said, "Man, did you have to tell me that?" but I was kind of glad she did. She warned me if I saw her after only an hour of the start of surgery, it meant they had closed my mother immediately because nothing could be done.

I couldn't blame Dr. Z. because I knew it hurt her to tell me, but it was not what I wanted to hear. I couldn't pass this information on to my family. That morning, we all arrived early with our hearts in our throats. As Mom was rolled down to the operating room, we were all by her side, trying hard to keep our tears from falling. Dad held her hand. We stayed while she signed zillions of forms, and doctors came to talk to her. They introduced themselves and told us what their roles in the procedure would be. When we saw Dr. Z and her partner, we knew it was time for her to go. Mom began to cry; I think we all did. Then, they took her away. It feels like you're watching them grow distant and then disappear before your very eyes, knowing that this might be for life or just an eternity of pain with no end in sight unless there is some sort miracle worker who can help make everything better. I'm sure many people feel like I did when my mom went into surgery that morning: scared and helpless because we had done all we could do but still didn't know how much longer she would live if at all…

Mom headed down to surgery at 6:30 a.m., and then we had to just hurry up and wait. Remember what Dr. Z told me? If I saw her within an hour of taking my mom down for surgery, it was because she could not be fixed. Roughly nine hours later and seventy days after the initial cancer diagnosis, Dr. Z and her partner showed up in the waiting room and told us to follow them into a family conference room. It was there that we heard the amazing words "optimally debulked!" They removed a fourteen-pound tumor along with other tumors too numerous to count. They fixed her hernia too. Cancer was found up to her diaphragm; that was part of the reason it had been so hard for her to eat. They took out her appendix and spleen, everything they could. Any microscopic stuff would be treated with "clean up" chemo. We all cried happy tears including Dr. Z. We were elated, relieved and could finally breathe for those moments.

My dad went home, and my sister and I waited to see her. It was my first time ever in an ICU; they'd made the decision to intubate Mom, which I found deeply unsettling. If you've ever had a loved one intubated, it's fucking terrifying. Our elation moments before turned to panic quickly when we entered the room. My sister and I almost passed out when we saw her after the surgery. She could not talk, but her eyes were open; we told her they had done it. *She* had done it. She was clean. All the cancer was gone.

Tears began streaming out of her eyes. Because of the tube down her throat, she could not talk. We sat and talked to her for a while, and suddenly alarms started going off, and people were rushing to her bedside. I swear, each fucking time we had a moment of positivity and hope, there was always some kind of negative tradeoff. At this point it had happened so many times it was as if whoever was in charge upstairs was really taking pleasure in fucking with us. So much had been taken out of her body that now she was reacting to the void inside her. It is not uncommon after a large surgery, if there is a lot of blood loss and a lot removed, for your body could go into shock. It is a medical emergency. Her blood pressure was sixty over twenty, and they had to flood her system with fluids.

Mom stayed in ICU for two days after the surgery and got discharged to the oncology floor on August 7th. Everyone told us Mom was "one tough cookie," and they were right. With the cancer removed, all the pressure was relieved, and she, too, could breathe again. Dr. Z. had not been confident before the surgery that they could optimally debulk her, but Mom stayed alive on the table, and they did a great job. We never do anything easy. Unfortunately, my mom's pathology showed exceedingly rare and deadly ovarian carcinosarcoma with heterologous elements, rhabdomyosarcomas, and chondroid and homologous elements leiomyosarcoma. I'll save you the trip to Google. "Ovarian cancer is the fifth leading cause of cancer-related death in women, with 22,280 cases and 15,500 deaths in 2012. The majority of ovarian cancers are epithelial tumors, the most common of which are serous carcinomas." (American Cancer Society)

My mom had ovarian carcinosarcomas, which are rare tumors composed of malignant epithelial and mesenchymal components. It is also called MMMT. Malignant, Mixed Mullerian Tumor. It is a very rare, aggressive cancer of the ovary and/or tissues of the female genital tract with characteristics of two types of cancer—carcinoma and sarcoma. It is associated with a poor outcome with a five-year survival rate of roughly 25%. "It is estimated that carcinosarcomas account for 1-4% of malignant ovarian cancers." (The National Center for Biotechnology Information.)

The only good part of the report was that all of her lymph nodes were clear; in addition to a small liver resection, they removed her appendix and took too many tumors to count off of her diaphragm. A lot of people do survive ovarian 3C, but would my mom have that kind of luck?

After extended post-op care, she was admitted to the hospital's inpatient rehab, the goal being for her to get up more independently and get physical and occupational therapy. Believe it or not, even after a huge nine-hour surgery like the one my mom went through, the medical protocol is to get the catheter out as soon as possible and get you up and out of bed.

Depending on the severity of the condition and pain management, it is usually only a couple days maximum before they get you up into a chair and/or using a commode or bedpan. Long term catheter use can cause infections, and the longer you do not get up, the harder it will be when you do. There are also many other risks, including blood clots. She had been gutted and needed to get back into shape to perform everyday living skills so she could go home. Do not forget she had been admitted nine days prior to surgery for TPN (IV nutrition), as she was malnourished and at surgical risk, so it was now almost a month she had been in the hospital.

As my mother's luck consistently demonstrated, I found the rehabilitation center's head to be quite the asshole. I am confident he did not read her chart or take the time to get to know my mom, her preexisting conditions, medical file, or history. Going through the medical file, I saw that it read: 68-year-old THIN BLACK FEMALE. No disrespect, but my mom is white. Typo?

She was hypotensive, had always had low blood pressure, and this doctor gave her meds for hypertension. Early in her stay, she called me to say she felt dizzy after she was placed on a new medication by the new Asshole Rehab Doctor. I asked her what it was, and thankfully, she knew it was a medicine for hypertension, aka high blood pressure.

I told her on the phone to stop taking the medication. As usual, things are not easy to manage unless you are there, so I got in my car and immediately drove to the inpatient rehab. I found the prescribing doctor and asked why he had her on hypertensive meds, and he pulled a white coat attitude with me. "I'm the doctor, I know what I'm doing, so basically, who the fuck are you?"

I told him my mom had called and said she was dizzy and had always been hypotensive, and I questioned him giving her high blood pressure medication. He was not interested in my questions, so I told him that if she fell because she was dizzy, he was 100 percent liable. I then left campus and drove to her cardiologist's office so I could get her on board to contact this rehab doctor and discontinue the medication that was putting her at risk of falling.

She never had a cardiologist before she was diagnosed with cancer. We discovered she was tachycardic at some point during this whole process. Going through her medical records years later, I found out she had had a heart attack no one had ever told us about. I had no appointment and told the receptionist that I needed to see the doctor. They looked at me like I had two heads, but I told them it was an emergency. She came into the waiting room, and I told her about the medication that the rehab doctor had put my mom on even though they were counter-indicated for her care. The cardiologist intervened and got her off those meds, but from then on, my mother and I both had a piss-poor attitude with the rehab doctor.

She did inpatient rehab for two weeks. If you have ever been in a hospital for a long time, you know that you really cannot sleep. You have no control over when people come in and out of your room. If it is not nurses giving meds, it is nursing aides or assistants taking vitals every hour. Lab technicians can be there a couple times a day, and they usually start before the sun comes up so they can have results for when the doctors begin to make rounds, which is usually around 8 am or before. Custodial services, food service, social workers, case workers, specialty services –you name it, they will be there. If you are in a teaching hospital, you can probably double the amount of people who will come into your room at any given time. As I said earlier, because Mom worked nights for forty years, she wasn't a morning person. Having someone knock on her door bright and early to do physical and occupational therapy was a nightmare for her.

When she was finally discharged on August 22nd, she'd been in the hospital for twenty-seven days—from not knowing when we would be able to schedule surgery on July 26th to discharge from inpatient rehab on August 22nd.

THINGS WE LEARNED IN AUGUST:

1.   White coat syndrome is a real thing. It is scientifically proven that people get "white coat hypertension" in hospitals or around doctors. Doctors are less likely to build long- term relationships with their patients; they may have too many cases and be overwhelmed. The constant news about medical errors can reduce trust in doctors and hospitals, which can frighten people away from care. The patient often does not question a doctor's direction because of the white coat. I cannot tell you how many times I have met people afraid to get second opinions who stick with one doctor their entire life. I am not saying that is always a bad choice; not all doctors are cocky assholes like the one we dealt with in in- patient rehab. As a patient, you are given patient rights, and those include the right to refuse care and medicine. If your loved one does not have the capacity or means to do that, it is your job to do it for them. As much as you love your ill family member, you must keep them in charge of their care, especially big decisions that could mean life or death.

When my mom proceeded with surgery, she was tired, weak, and spent. Nothing had worked in her favor, but the next steps had to be her decision and her decision alone. We told her we would stand by whatever her decision was, even if it hurt. As much as surgeons can come off very matter-of-fact and clinical, I do think that they do care. Most of the providers my mom had did care about her. That does not mean they did not fuck up; it means that I think they cared about her but were sloppy. At the end of the day—and I have learned this myself—, you want a good mechanic to fix your car. You want an expert who is great at their specialty. Dr. Z and her colleague were excellent at both bedside manner and their surgical craft.

Bedside manner refers most often to the way a medical professional interacts with patients. A doctor with a good bedside manner demonstrates empathy and emits an aura of ease for the patients, while also involving them in health decisions. It is really a toss-up what you will get on any given day with your doctor and/or their team. For the most part you hope you do not get someone who is rude, dismissive, and has a cold attitude. It is better to have a relationship, but when you are dealing with cancer or severe, acute illness and hospitalized a lot, you will likely get both. It is just a numerical certainty. As an advocate, you must be there to fight the rude ones who may not be listening or do not see any error in their orders. When my mom was in rehab, she was given medicine to slow her heart rate down in error. Her heart rate was already on the slow side, so this could have made her pass out or worse. Thankfully, she was aware enough to know and tell me. The prescribing doctor took no responsibility or feedback until I got the medical specialist involved to discontinue the medicine. What if she had not told me? What if she had fallen and hit her head on the floor or worse?

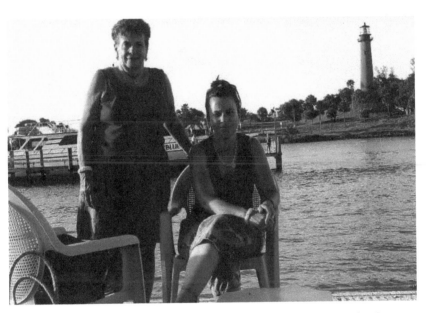

My mom and me in Florida. My sister and my nephews went to Florida
or South Carolina every summer until my mom got sick.

6

SEPTEMBER

My mom was home for a couple of days, and on Thursday, September 2nd, they were going to start the cleanup chemo. This had to be done inpatient, one round a day, four full treatments. The first day she had it, she was okay. The second day she had it, I got an email from my sister while I was at work with the subject line: "Fucking terrible." I started Googling the chemo treatment they were using, and it had nitrogen mustards—a product derived from chemical nerve gases like Agent Orange. I know the point of chemo is to kill cells, but still, holy shit. I went over to the hospital with my printout in hand, and she had every symptom of toxicity (poisoning) except for coma and death. She was hallucinating, barely conscious, and looked dead in the bed. We had been told these rounds of chemo would be easy, that they would be nothing like the shit we dealt with before.

Her oncologist was off campus, so I drove to his office. It was around 5:30 pm on the Friday of Labor Day weekend; he had a boat, and I knew I needed to catch him before he took off and was unreachable. I made him come to the hospital and take a look at Mom. He said, "She's fine. This is normal. We're going for the cure, and we have to get through this." I told him that I had looked up her medication and symptoms of toxicity, and I thought she was toxic that night. He disagreed and told me to stay off the internet. My mom liked Dr. X and trusted him, so we agreed to do another round of chemo. My sister and I stayed with her, and my mom went to sleep.

Saturday morning, the nurse called me on my cell when she started her shift on the oncology floor. We had spent so much time on this hospital floor, the nurses all knew us by now. Remember, I told you that it is critical you get to know your RNs, LVNs, nursing assistants, and charge nurses, and this is the case in point. Nurses are the connective tissue at the hospital; they are the ones who see the patient enough to know when something is wrong. This nurse hadn't seen Mom for a couple of weeks, and when she did see her, she said, "What the hell happened to Connie?"

During the call, one of the charge nurses said she had orders to hang another bag (chemo treatment), but she wouldn't do it until we got there. My sister, father, and I all rushed over to the hospital. I found my mother lying flat on her back, arm dangling off the bed. She looked so weak and helpless that it broke my heart. Vomit leaked from between unwilling lips as she lay there, speechless, in pain, with no one willing or able to help her. This is not something any person should ever have go through alone; I will do everything possible to make sure this never happens again. Do you know how many cancer patients die of choking on their own vomit? This was my mother, the same lady who polished her shoes every morning before she left the house for work, and she was lying there lifeless, helpless, covered in her own puke. Strike FUCKING 4, I was irate. Dr. X was already gone for the weekend, so we had to get one of his partners to see her.

This is another problem with healthcare today; you have these large groups, medical Wal-Marts, and the "on calls" don't know you. They don't know what you look like when you're in pain, when you're okay, how you smile, your affect, nothing. You are just a folder, a case, another patient. This on-call partner from oncology said, again, "Hang tough, she's going to be okay. We're going for the cure." My mother forced one eye open and agreed to just get this over with. We couldn't leave that night; she was hallucinating, and every time she moved her head, she vomited. I did not trust anybody anymore; we stayed with her, afraid that she would aspirate on her own vomit if we left. She did the fourth and last round of chemo; it could not be over fast enough.

September 5th was the last round, and the next day, the 6th, she weighed in at 119 pounds. She was constantly nauseated and already filling up with ascites again. They took her for X-rays to make sure the "umbrellas" were working, and there were no clots; she threw up every time she moved or opened her eyes. When Dr. X returned from the long weekend, on Tuesday, September 7th, I was at the entrance of her room. He stopped, looked at me, and said very fucking calmly, "You were right. She is toxic."

I understand oncology is probably one of the hardest professions you can be in; it's science, but it's also art. I also know that every patient an oncologist treats is different and may experience their ordered treatments differently. I understand that unlike in many other medical specialties, an oncologist is often tasked with the very tough job of telling their patient that they have a life-changing and possibly life-ending disease that has no treatment guarantees, success rates, or survival rates. But—and this is a big fucking but—I just Googled her symptoms and knew she was toxic. It was his goddamn job. It was his specialty, his orders, his advice, his back up, his error.

My poor mom suffered for two weeks from being poisoned. I had to call my husband three times in those two weeks to leave work because we thought she would not make it. My family was there around the clock because my mom was so sick that we thought she would die at any second. My mom had very little color in her face, and she wasn't even moving anymore. She would slip out of consciousness for several seconds before coming back and opening an eye or giving us a slight movement that let us all know she was still with us. Our spirits sunk as days turned into weeks without word about what treatment plan might work best against this terrible disease. My sister, my dad, and I were on autopilot at this point, and, because there was absolutely no trust, we juggled our schedules to try to make sure there was always one of us there when the doctors made rounds, during the day and at night before visiting hours were over. About every 48 hours during this period, my mom had to keep having the ascites drained.

Why was the ascites coming back with such vengeance? We had gotten all the cancer out, right? This was "clean up" chemo for the leftover microscopic cancer they could not get during a nine-hour surgery.

But if something could go wrong at this point, it was going to go wrong.

It is not uncommon to see a priest on the oncology floor. In the weeks following the cleanup chemo, he came into my mother's room four times. I appreciate having a priest around, but I did not want to see him in my mother's room. We are not deeply religious, and when you see that white- collar at the door, it freaks you out. My mother might have had private conversations with him, but needing a priest was not part of our plan.

Unfortunately, after becoming toxic, any giddy up she had in her step, any optimism after the debulking, was gone. The poisoning and the suffering and fright that came with it just knocked the wind out of her sails. During this two-week period, I called Anthony twice at work in New York City to come to the hospital. All the signals were saying she was not going to come out of this poisoning. As my dad tried to keep a stiff upper lip, sometimes I saw them having private moments in her room, and I saw them crying. My dad was trying to be strong, but fuck, this was killing all of us. My sister, usually, was the one who was able to bring any positivity to the situation. This is not to say she was not aware of how bad things were, but she managed to hide her emotions better than my dad and I did.

Toward the end of the weeks following her toxicity, Mom had other visitors like her brothers, my aunts, and close family friends. She didn't want visitors per say, but this gives you an idea of how bad things were.

I hope if you are reading this, you never find yourself on an oncology floor. But according to the American Cancer Society, in

2020, roughly 1.8 million people will be diagnosed with cancer in the United States. An estimated 606,520 people will die from cancer in the same year; this equates to roughly 1,662 people dying of cancer each day in 2020.

Before she was discharged, they wanted to do a scan because her blood levels were off again, and the ascites was also back. On September 13th, she had a CAT scan of her abdomen and pelvis with contrast. As our luck would have it, the fucking cancer was back with a vengeance. Sometimes, you think to yourself, 'How the fuck can it possibly get worse?' And then, bam! It does.

Her CAT scan impression read: consistent with surgery but marked tumor progression with extensive intraperitoneal tumor on the abdomen and pelvis. Anasarca and worsened atelectasis in the right lower lobe with pleural effusion. Large amounts of ascites, marked tumors, one is 8.3x5.9 cm. .

The CAT actually says that the tumors are worse than the CAT before the surgery; "marked worsening since 7/2/10."

Forty days post-op and more cancer than we started with. They now knew that this chemo regimen was toxic, and they could not use it on my mom. "Recurring" ovarian cancer sometimes can be treated with Doxil, so that was our last resort. It was considered a maintenance/quality of life decision. They said, "It keeps the disease at bay" and stops it from growing. We were out of options, so this was going to be it.

September 20th, discharge notes: "68-year-old woman with carcinosarcoma, status post optimal debulking, who was admitted her first cycle and cisplatin. At the time of her surgery, she was deemed optimally debulked. (Codeword "we got everything except lingering microscopic cells and/ or tumors less than 2 cm in size.") She received systemic chemotherapy without incident initially with some slight nausea. Towards the end of the 4-day infusion, the patient began having some mental status changes and increasing somnolence. Also, in this period, she received paracentesis three times for recurrent ascites." Here is where I want to punch someone right in the mouth: "It was felt that at the end of her infusion, she was suffering from ifosfamide toxicity."

Really? That is your discharge report, when I told you on day one of chemo that she was toxic, and I'm not a professional? "Towards the end of day four infusion, the patient began having some mental status changes and increasing somnolence."

BULLSHIT! This stole my mother's time; stole her spirit, and I think in my heart of hearts, finding out the cancer returned destroyed any remaining hope we had. I can't blame her. We did not know the phrase "give up." We just kept on going with the "Keep on fighting" speeches and positive vibes, but all the time, she was suffering for us. FUCK!

THINGS WE LEARNED IN SEPTEMBER:

1. There is a reason why doctors and hospitals must carry medical malpractice insurance. They are human and make mistakes. While you should not try to take their role because you are not qualified, there will be times that you need to question their decision-making, especially if it has to do with a very sick loved one or yourself. Trust your instincts. What if the amazing nurse who was worried about how bad my mom looked had not called me and had instead just proceeded with the doctor's orders as scheduled? What if we hadn't had the relationship with the nurses that gave this nurse the courage and tenacity to feel secure to call me on my cell? What if I had not gone as soon as the nurse called me? Would my mom have aspirated? This poisoning was completely negligent, and it robbed us of the little hope we had left.

The internet can be your worst enemy or your best friend. It depends on how you use it and how good you are at fact-finding when it is crucial. From my experience, I can tell you it did create a lot of false hope for me initially, but it also connected me to resources, groups, and alternative options for my mom's care, including holistic supplements. Doing a basic Google search on her "clean up" chemo gave me the information I needed to see that my mom was toxic. She had every symptom except coma and death. Use it wisely. You have an abundance of information at your fingertips that is generally very easy to get. Still, while you should research your illness, medication, side effects, etc., your medical team should be the lead in this area. You could wind up driving your medical team crazy with incorrect information and not realize it is old or there are new studies out there you are not privy to that conflict with your findings. You have to allow them to lead, but dammit, as Ronald Reagan said, "Trust but verify."

You can make excuses or you can make it happen.

Do not take "No" for an answer.

7

OCTOBER

id-October, she was feeling a little better. After they came clean with us about how the cleanup chemo had poisoned her, Dr. Z suggested that we put her on Doxil, maintenance chemotherapy. She would probably be on it for the rest of her life, but it wasn't a hard treatment, and she could live with it. It was a plan to keep her alive, manage the ascites, and keep whatever was growing in her at bay. It was not an inpatient thing or an all-day in the chemo suite thing; Doxil is used for many different cancers.

Two steps forward, five steps back—at this point, why would anything go our way? On October 6th, she had her first outpatient Doxil treatment. She was so depressed and not really eating, just trying her best for us. On October 21st, my mom also decided that because she had two daughters, she would get tested for the BRCA gene. There are two phases, but she only had the first, because it came back negative.

Based on the four types of carcinomas the pathology report

showed after the debulking surgery she had, I don't think my mother could have been saved. The cancer was rare and lethal. She continued to go to the oncologist for blood work, and my sister tried to pair visits with paracentesis. They pulled her CA125 level to see what range it was in, white blood cell count, platelet count; everything was within normal limits, or if not, at least it wasn't way out of whack.

Her mind was not good, though; she was defeated, being the designated hitter in this shit game was getting harder every inning. Every time I went to her house, I found her in bed. Just getting her to sit outside for a half hour was like pulling teeth. She had every reason to be acutely depressed, but I pushed her; I brought her manicotti, green drinks, sweets, holistic mushrooms, everything I could think of. I had read about holistic mushrooms that were supposed to be magical cure-alls. They tasted like dirt, and she never ate them. The emails I sent to my sister were all stories about patients who had been debulked but had recurring cancer.

Everyone tried to help. The living room was lined with cards from everyone, and people stopped by when she allowed them. Some of her close friends did not visit, but called. I'm not sure if this was my mom's choice or theirs, but she was tired—beaten down and dealing with her own mortality. Some relatives did not come because they had a very hard time seeing my mom in the condition that she was in. It's not fucking easy seeing someone you love waste away mentally and physically, getting weaker, withdrawn, and more ill with each passing day.

In retrospect, I don't blame them. I did then. I was pissed at some people I thought should have made a fucking effort, but who was I to make that demand? Realistically, this was to satisfy my own expectations, and if you were to ask my mom, she would have probably preferred to avoid the uncomfortable visits.

Everyone means well, don't get me wrong, but you run out of things to say. At this point, the cancer was the gun, and it was fully loaded with one in the chamber. These decisions are not easy and, in the end, everyone deals with this shit differently.

As a Hail Mary, I found an exclusive cancer treatment center in Pennsylvania called the Cancer Treatment Center of America. Their pitch is treating the entire mind, body and soul with both Eastern and Western medicine They would have taken her, but Mom would not go. I knew it was probably a "no" we were all desperate for something to help, anything, because every day that passed, things got worse.

My birthday was on October 27th. I turned forty, and we went out to a local hibachi restaurant to celebrate with my nephews and my uncles (all October birthdays). She ate a little bit. My father was trying to make jokes and drinking shots of sake. My mother gave me a note and seagull earrings that had belonged to my grandmother. That was the last time she ever ate out; I'm not sure if she ever went out in public at all after that. Looking back at that night, it was a big deal for my mom to get dressed and try to put on a smile to celebrate birthdays in public when she was so sick. During dinner, we all saw the writing on the wall, but nobody was talking about it.

We laughed and ate while everyone passed Luke around the table, because even though we were at hibachi, the fire antics of the chef got old quickly to an energetic toddler. For those couple hours, we were able to escape from reality and live in blissful ignorance of what was really going on and the ugly future we all knew lay ahead.

When we were leaving, we had to walk by the bar; my mother, bald and obviously sick, was holding onto my father's arm, and this group of twenty-somethings just wouldn't get out of the way. Of course, we were hypersensitive to it, and my husband, a former Marine who was born in the Bronx, said, "You better get the fuck out of the way before I move you."

Trust me: they moved.

At least Mom made it out for my birthday one last time. During this month, my mom continued getting paracentesis roughly every two to three days because the dam ascites just would not let up. The amount of fluid they removed on each visit varied from four liters to as high as seven. It really depended on how many days went by in between treatments. This was no way to live.

THINGS WE LEARNED IN OCTOBER:

1. Sometimes, no matter how much you try, follow the rules, be a good person in life, the deck is stacked against you. There are things we can control and things that we can't, and being in a fight for your life for six long months and continually being knocked down is exhausting. It will impact your mental health. It is essential to keep a positive outlook on things because there is the mind/body connection, but you also must have realistic expectations for the one in the fight and for their future. At this point on our ride through hell, I know my mom was just going through the motions for us. She was mentally and physically drained. Doxil was our last hope, and looking back, it really just prolonged my mom's suffering.

2. Be as supportive as you can, but remind your loved one that they are in charge of their treatment decisions and life choices. While nobody wants to ever lose a loved one, sometimes watching someone suffer is worse than letting them go in peace.

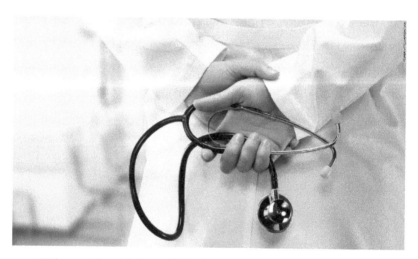

"Clean up chemo," they said. "No big deal." Always trust your instincts.

8

NOVEMBER

At this time, my mom was not feeling well at all, physically or mentally. She had a lot of back pain, and the ascites and the need for paracentesis would not give her a break. My sister took her multiple times a week for relief from this horrible fluid. This way of life and the need for this procedure was frustrating, depressing, and exhausting. She had her second Doxil treatment on November 3rd. They also gave her Lasix and made her wear compression stockings because of all of the fluid she was retaining. We may not have wanted to say it out loud, but all signs at this point were bad. For example, on the ninth they tapped (paracentesis) her and took 6.3 liters out; two days later, they took out five liters. At this point, the chemo wasn't doing anything. She was just weak, requiring paracentesis almost every other day, losing weight and not eating, and sleeping most of the day. She had fallen a couple of times and not told us about it. I think she knew that death was imminent. I didn't want to know; I didn't want it to be that way, but we all told my mother from the beginning she was in charge of her healthcare choices. Unfortunately for her, we were always in the red. All things being equal, nobody should have to experience these horrible things. But all of us do, at some point or another. It is just when and how bad.

We knew Doxil was a hail Mary. I think my mom was done when Dr. Z told us forty days after being optimally debulked that the cancer was back and there was more on the scan than there had been to begin with. She did the Doxil for us. On November 17th, she had an oncologist visit, and she was very weak and dehydrated. They scheduled a CAT scan of her abdomen and pelvis with contrast for the next day. The fucking cancer was everywhere. On November 19th, she had paracentesis again, and they removed four liters. November 25th was Thanksgiving.

My sister brought Thanksgiving down to my parent's house, and I had pneumonia, so of course I couldn't be around a cancer patient. She probably slept through most of it anyway, but I was really upset to not be able to be there.

Of all the fucking times to get sick, I had to get sick now. I practically lived in the hospital for six months, and now I had to get something bad enough that I couldn't be around my mom. Seriously, what the fuck?

On November 26th, she had paracentesis for the last time. We had to come to grips with the fact that treatment was not working; cancer had dug in, and nothing was helping.

On Saturday, November 27th, we had a hospice intake nurse come to my parents' house for her care interview. The role of the hospice nurse is to focus **solely on end-of-life care,** either in a facility or in the patient's home. Not only do they manage pain and other symptoms, they assist in the process of death with dignity. We were all in my parents living room, my mom on the couch sitting up. She did not want to die in the hospital, and we did not want her to die alone. She was coherent and mindful of her choices. It was a heart-ripping discussion, but we had to stand strong and support my mom's decision to stop treatment. Nothing was working, and she was suffering.

My God, was she suffering.

Cognitively, she was probably in the best shape I had seen her in in a very long time; she wasn't lethargic or tired or depressed. My mom was almost—I do not want to say at peace because she didn't want to leave—but she had finally reached a point where she could hang up her jacket and say, "Okay, I'm done."

When the lady interviewed her, she was on point about everything; she answered all the questions correctly, and she knew all the medication she was on and was very clear. When the nurse, left we all sat silent, sort of numb. My Dad went outside to "find" work to be done to keep himself busy as he did for months and still does to this day. My sister and I tried to go about any normal routine at the house even though we were both fucking dying inside.

On November 30th, they gave my mom a pain patch, but she didn't like it because it made her hallucinate. They gave her an oxygen tank, but she didn't use it at first. This was the last day she ate anything, and she began seeing my grandmother, talking to her and hallucinating.

THINGS WE LEARNED IN NOVEMBER:

1.	Adjust your priorities. My mom's illness caught us off guard. My dad had had heart disease, lifesaving heart surgery, and three and a half stents due to congestive heart failure five years prior to my mom getting sick. Statistically and realistically, he had a hell of a lot more problems than my mom seemed to. As you read earlier, this started with indigestion. Unfortunately, my mom self-treated, and because of fear, she did not seek out care earlier. Given her pathology, I don't think that would have changed the outcome, but it may have. So many people from my mom's generation (they are called the Silent Generation) are not proactive with self- care. The Silent Generation is made up of those born from 1925 to 1945 —because they were raised during a period of war and economic depression. The label reflects the counterculture of a rebellious generation, distrustful of the establishment and keen to find their own voice. The definition is pretty on point, at least based on what I have observed with other family and friends.

Make time, make memories, and don't put stuff off too far into the future. Before the phone call I got on May 1st, life was excellent. I had a baby, a good career, a happy family, and lots of love. There are things I wish I had done differently. I chose to work during her illness for many reasons, but I wish I had had more time. Even if she was sick, I wish I had had more time, more meaningful conversations, and peace. I felt like most of those months were reactive, putting fires out and in constant worry and anxiety. I see peers today who still have both parents and don't make time, talk negatively about them, see them as a "pain"; they really do not realize what they have and how lucky they are. It pisses me off.

2.   Healthcare is a complex universe. We, as humans, need doctors. Doctors need patients. But sometimes, particularly with cancer, you need to trust your gut. They are not magicians. They are not superheroes. There is a limit to what they can do for you. I am empathetic to the job of an oncologist. While I remain angry at my mom's, I have educated myself on their jobs and patient interactions, responsibilities, blame they take, second guessing, and sometimes impossible expectations that they get from families.

3.   There is a limit to what the human body can withstand, tolerate, and recover from. You never want to lose hope, but you have to find a way to be realistic when the end has come. It is the patient's choice, and no matter how much it hurts, you have so support them. My mom suffered every fucking day from May 1st on. Nothing was working. The doctors threw everything at it, and she stayed in the game into overtime, but it was time to call it. She wasn't afraid. She just worried about us. Each of us told her it was okay to go, and that is important. Nothing prepares you for these kinds of situations. There's no dress rehearsal.

9

DECEMBER

By Wednesday, December 1st, Mom was significantly less responsive; she was very weak and dehydrated; the hospice people were coming every day to check on her. They were using a syringe to administer morphine; she was almost unconscious, but still a little alert. Mom slept on the couch, and I would sit in the living room and watch her stomach go up and down to make sure she was still breathing. One day, one of the hospice ladies was on the phone with her people ordering more morphine, and I heard her tell them to hurry, because, "This one's going down fast." She's lucky I didn't knock her out right in the kitchen.

This one's going down fast.

Right in front of me she said this. I get it; they become numb to it, but are you fucking kidding me? We didn't complain, (although I told hospice afterward and they were mortified) but I just could not have another fight on my hands right then. From the day my mom signed up for hospice care, my sister and I slept at my parents' house.

We didn't leave because we didn't know when we were going to lose her.

My sister and I were talking and even though we didn't want her to go, we wondered if maybe she wouldn't pass if we were there. We wondered if we should leave for an hour or so. But then, we didn't want to leave, because we didn't want to not be there. It's just so many fucked up feelings that you go through. Even having the conversation was fucking sad, and it still makes me feel riddled with guilt almost ten years later. We were giving her the morphine, and once, I accidentally gave her ten milligrams instead of five. When I realized what I had done, at first, I was upset, and then I wondered if it would be better if the morphine did slow down Mom's nervous system until it stopped. Maybe I would have done her a favor? This is a dark example of the headspace you find yourself in when watching someone die. Nothing short of torture.

At this point my sister, my dad, and I were there most of the time. Anthony and Todd (my sister's husband) were also there when they weren't working. Anthony also had Luke with him, but it was really no place for a toddler. We were all emotionally and physically spent. My dad passed the time working outside, and my sister and I just walked in circles around the house. We each spent individual time with my mom, both when she was alert and not alert. As she lay motionless on the couch, I was caught in a hundred-yard stare in the chair, watching her chest rise and fall. It's a fucked up thing being with someone when they die. You stand guard to make sure they are breathing, but ultimately you are waiting for them to stop.

If you have never been through it, it is absolutely fucking

horrifying. I remember holding her hand and telling her it was okay to go. She was so fucking skinny. Her hand was riddled with rheumatoid arthritis, and it just lay in mine. Sometimes, I might get a squeeze or a finger movement, and for a brief second, it would wake me up from my hopeless emotion. I told her I loved her and hugged her. We all did. I'm sure—in fact, I know—that my parents had many additional conversations about these moments that my sister and I did not know, but that was okay, because that was their special bond.

We had three different hospice ladies. Every day, the hospice nurses check the patient's breathing and pulse, check their ankles, feet, and hands for inflammation, and every day they say, "Today is going to be the day."

They said that for a week.

On the last day the woman who came was the midwife who had delivered both my nephews. I don't think any of us knew she also worked for hospice, so it was nice to see a familiar face

My sister, her husband, my dad, and I were there, and I told Anthony to take Luke home. I figured there was no need for him to stay because we could not do anything.

Don't forget my parents' home is 900 square feet, so even though we may have been in different rooms, we were all in close proximity to the living room and my mom on the couch at all times.

I remember it like it was yesterday; my sister noticed the labored breathing and a gurgle. When people pass, they get this gurgle; they call it the death rattle, and my mother's breathing became very labored the evening of December 4th. We called my dad out of the bedroom, and we all hugged her and cried and told her we loved her, and it was okay to go. Leave this fucking world of pain and suffering in peace. My sister, her husband, and I went into the kitchen and my dad sat with her on the couch. She had a moment of clarity and said to him, "We were supposed to grow old together." My father told her it was okay, he cried, and soon after, she stopped breathing. He shut her eyes, and we were all in shock although we had been waiting for this moment for an entire week.

I really don't remember much except I called my husband to return to my parent's house, since he had just left and was only about ten minutes away. We called the coroner who, coincidentally, we had also gone to high school with. We wrapped my mom in a blanket, and Anthony went outside with them to make sure they were gentle and respectful with her. He, too, was emotional, but it is just in him to be a protector, and he knew that none of us were in the shape to go outside.

The rest of us were in the house, shell-shocked. It fucked me up. After midnight, I sent an email telling my friends what had happened. My best friend Leslie lived in the same town and came and sat on my parents' steps for a while, not knowing what to do, until finally she came inside. It was one in the morning. That is what you call a fucking friend. That is what you call a ride or die. That is someone who had no idea what she was walking into and came anyway. My dad was also very moved that she came; she walked into a really bad, heavy and emotionally charged situation to support us, without hesitation. I will never forget that. She is still, to this day, my rock.

As luck would have it, and why not add to the bucket of fucks that were given throughout this entire ordeal, the bigger hospice long term supplies arrived the day after Mom died. I think my dad made the phone call to quickly get them picked up and out of there.

We had Mom cremated; she didn't want to be laid out. She always said she didn't want people looking at her when she was dead. She didn't have a mean bone in her body, so while my thoughts were aligned, they were a little harsher than hers were. My thoughts were, 'If you don't come see me when I'm alive don't' bother to come when I'm dead.'

We had a local priest do a little mass; we held a wake from 2 p.m. to 4 p.m. and 7 p.m. to 9 p.m., and he came in around 8:30 p.m. My father had been a firefighter for forty years, so there were lots of firefighters there, family, friends, her customers, bingo buddies, and many people from my office; the place was packed. In the morning, we had a memorial service, and I wrote my speech fifteen minutes before I left the house. My Meyers Briggs is ENFP, so procrastination is my specialty, but some of my best writing or projects have been done under stress and against the clock. I managed not to cry until the end, and yes, I was eating Xanax. Of course, my sister had hers prepared well in advance with music.

The firehouse had a reception after the service where they served food and let us all gather. These gatherings are fucked up. You already got all the "I'm sorrys" at the funeral parlor and cemetery, so then, I guess it is supposed to be the time that your loved ones, family, and friends gather to celebrate the life lost. Personally? I hated it. Every fucking second of it. Because it was taking everything out of me to not curl up in a ball in a corner somewhere and hide from everyone. This was the final act, the curtain was drawn, we had lost the game, and it wasn't even close. My tank was empty, but I still had to socialize because that was what was expected. I also had Luke, so he made it bearable. Chasing him around kept my mind off the reality of the situation.

I bought eight little jars and took some of her ashes. I have some here at my house and some in a necklace. Some people have the ashes put into the ink for a tattoo, but I don't think I'm quite ready for that. I had my mother's gravestone made by some guy in New Jersey; it's an angel holding a heart, and now there are three others in the cemetery like it. It's beautiful. I have two tattoos on my back for her; one is an angel and the other a fairy. I still have to finish them. Hopefully this year.

THINGS WE LEARNED IN DECEMBER:

1.   It was only a week, but the week of hospice felt like a month. We never wanted to be in this place, but when we found out that the cancer had returned, it was kind of inevitable. My poor mom had fought the fight, endured all the ups and downs, side effects, possible complications, medical mistakes, and any hope of beating this lousy fucking disease was gone. She was weak, very sick, and mentally prepared for her mortality.

2.   Sometimes, the best planning does not go as expected. Each day after the hospice intake, the hospice staff who visited the house said, "Today will be the day." She lived Saturday to Saturday. Seven days of "It will be today" and it wasn't. It wasn't their fault; they only share what they think by looking at the patient, but I almost wish they wouldn't say it with such guarantee or confidence. They have a very hard job, so it is difficult to be judgmental, but this was our first time using such a service. If I had to do it all over again, I would ask more questions. For example, how long has the staff been providing hospice service? Do they specialize in any illness, say, cancer? Are there limits on what treatment they can provide? We didn't know that there would be three different staff members, and what time they would be arriving, so it would have been good if we had known that in advance. Not that we were busy doing anything else, but having and knowing

that a second head and trained opinion was coming to look at my mom was already stressful. Knowing what time or having a better schedule and consistency in staff would have made it easier.

10

THE NEW NORMAL

As I said at the beginning of this book, after my mom passed, I was convinced I didn't need to speak to anyone even though I had DSM V textbook acute depression, anxiety, and PTSD. I finally started talking to somebody about it. Still, it took a long time for me to be able to have the conversation. It's better now, but it took a while. It made me a bitch, it made me self-destructive, and it made me despondent and angry. I wonder all the time if there's something we could have done differently that would have changed the outcome for my mother. I think about Kathy Bates, the famous actress who was diagnosed with the same kind of cancer and stage. She had the surgery right away and survived and is still alive today. What if we had gotten the shit out quicker? What if this, what if that? My mother told me once: "Don't be foolish like me. Take care of your body. Take care of yourself. She had such guilt for not seeing a doctor all those years. She had just seen the Dr. Oz episode about ovarian cancer, and even though we told her she was being ridiculous, she knew from the beginning what was going on. I think the first doctor in the Emergency Room knew right then and there. I think that Dr. Cool knew, even though he gave us hope that it could be benign. You could see it in his face.

My sister found my mother's journal after she passed, and she had already written out what she wanted for a funeral in May. May! We weren't "officially" diagnosed until the end of May, and this was dated before that. She knew, but mentally, she felt so guilty and was worried about us. I think she went through the motions for her family. I think she had private conversations with Dr. Z that we did not know about. I think she did a lot for us and her grandchildren, but she always knew the result would not be what we wanted.

Throughout her illness, my sister, Alicia, and I were tight and cohesive; she had the hard job of being mom to my eight and twelve-year-old nephews. She did this while providing care for Luke while I worked and took my mom to many of her medical appointments. I was lucky because my sister was in a position to take care of Luke, and she was family. I think any mother would rather pay a family member to care for their child than a stranger. My mom did not really get the chance to know my son. He was fifteen months when she died. This makes me very sad because he will never know how much he missed.

We did everything as a family throughout her illness. After Mom was gone, my father needed a lot of paperwork and book keeping help; my mom did everything in that department. My dad is old school. My sister started helping with bills when Mom got sick, and she wanted to keep that role. She has it to this day. I cleaned up the medical bills. Again, because it was a teaching hospital, I had about an inch of invoices from names I did not recognize. Some were residents, random specialists who may have had a 5-minute consult, and everyone in between. While my parents had good insurance, there were still plenty of bills the hospital and various medical groups were looking for payment on. I wasn't in any rush to pay them.

After my mom died, I wanted to litigate; I wanted my pound of flesh. What I didn't want was money. It was about teaching them a fucking lesson. There had been too many errors on their watch. While my mom was very sick, she suffered at their hand due to incompetence and lack of communication. My father and sister didn't want to do it, though.

I didn't want to fight with them about it, but I wanted blood. I decided to write a letter to the CEO of the hospital, because responsibility is at the top. You have all heard the saying, "Shit rolls downhill." I told him that I was not going to litigate, but I also informed him of five of roughly 25 fuck-ups that happened because of his staff and asked him to zero balance my parents' net bill of roughly $5,000.00. Two weeks later I received a letter that they had zero balanced my parents' account. The CEO must have had to sit in a room with so many attorneys, because by zero balancing the bill he admitted guilt and liability. He needed to know what had happened on his watch; my mother was a very sick woman who suffered needlessly because of these fuck-ups. He had a choice; it could have been $10,000,000, or whatever number was worked up, or $5,000.00. I had an attorney look at her records, and I did have a malpractice case. To me, it should have been an easy decision for him to make considering I was giving him a choice. While I was happy, they zero balanced my parents account, I still did not feel whole. I felt cheated and angry.

I don't think I ever will forgive certain doctors, but money is meaningless in this case. It will not bring my mom back, it will not make her suffering disappear, it will not clear them of their sometimes-reckless liability. However, they did make changes because of my mother's case. After the surgery, when she had the cleanup chemo, the nurses did rounds every hour. After I found my mother on her back, when she could have aspirated on her own vomit, they changed that to every fifteen minutes if you were getting acute chemo in that hospital.

Another change was interdisciplinary case meetings. My family and I spent a whole lot of time with my mom. They held multidisciplinary weekly or biweekly case meetings, and the family was never included. I've seen my mother not want to hit the call button because she didn't want to bother the nurses. I've seen her unable to ambulate to the bathroom; I've seen her pass up meal after meal and just drink half a Boost instead. They didn't track her intake at all. If you're really sick and need to eat, food services just take your tray, and the nurses and doctors do not know if you have eaten. When you have cancer and wasting disease, your food intake is very important. I'm not blaming food services; it's just how the system works. In the letter, I basically said, "I may not be your best friend, but there are a lot of things you should know that the family can offer you to treat the whole patient. If there are ten minutes at the beginning of the meeting in which the family can rattle off mental health issues, symptoms, medication compliance, finances, whatever, just to give you a window into whatever's going on to help you treat the patient better, you should do that." So, they've changed that and now they include the family in these interdisciplinary meetings.

My mom is not the only person this has happened to. It happens every day. Everybody loses people. Doctor-patient relationships have gotten more detached in the ten years since my mother passed; now, so much of it happens online. If people can take away some of the lessons that I learned through these experiences, I'll be grateful. Sometimes you need to turn on the ugly side of you.

So, my adventures in the fucked-up world of health care continued after my mother passed, but I've wanted to write this book since she died ten years ago. Families understand maybe half the things you need to be thinking about when a loved one is critically ill. Insurance companies need to rethink shit; doctors and practitioners need to think about how they treat patients. If I can help families gain insight and share some lessons learned so their loved ones don't have to suffer the way my mother suffered, then that's all I want. It will preserve my mother's memory and help people think about the right way to do things. Ask a second time, get a second opinion, ask about the medication, and know your rights as a patient and a patient caregiver. You need to be there and if you can't be, get somebody else to be there.

Respect the nurses and treat them well, but you can't necessarily trust the staff wholly, because human error happens. I once walked into my mother's room and found that her IV hadn't been turned on all day; she hadn't been receiving the fluids she desperately needed to stay hydrated. It was pure human error.

I wrote this book to help educate people on how they can better advocate for their loved ones when there's a medical crisis or a prolonged illness, but nothing I say will help anyone if they're afraid to speak up on behalf of that loved one. Don't be afraid of people thinking you're difficult; don't be afraid to have a mouth and use your voice. Speak up and make sure that your loved one gets the help they need to survive. Their life depends on you.

Don't wait to have those conversations. Many families don't talk about their feelings until there is a crisis. Tell people you love them, and show it before it is too late. We went from returning from fun at the beach one day to the horror and worry of a possible cancer diagnosis in 24 hours. Life can change quickly, so try to enjoy it. Be grateful for what you have, and make memories.

11

TODAY

It's August 2021 as I sit here on my seventh edit of this book, and I still have a pit in my gut. After going through this again, rechecking all her medical records, reading how much my mom suffered brings me great sadness, but I'm grateful to share her story with the world. It is too important to me to not get right.

I've been lucky and received guidance from some smart people who pushed more out of my drafts, and I think this is it. Who would have thought our healthcare system would be in the state that it is in today in a 20-month pandemic global setting. As a New Yorker, I've seen the strain on many healthcare providers. I've talked to many who suffer from PTSD, because they were the connective tissue between dying loved ones and death—during a pandemic, you cannot have visitors. While this is a long and still unfolding subject, patient advocacy is more important now that it was 20 months ago.

Today, as I close this book for my last edit, many hospitals require loved ones to either be vaccinated or be COVID-negative to visit their loved ones. There are exceptions that can be made by the medical staff, but trust me when I say that this places more burden on the staff and fuels the climate for medical errors.

I myself was hospitalized during the end of 2020. My husband dropped me off with my son around 7:30 pm, and I was throwing up and in terrible agony. Neither my husband nor my son could stay in the emergency room or waiting room. In one way, it was good because I was so bad that I did not want my son seeing me that way. In another, it was bad because I know my husband would never have allowed me to wait seven hours before anyone actually decided to take me seriously.

I'll spare you the details, but I was bleeding internally. Half of the blood that belonged in my body was in my stomach. The Physician Assistant looked down my throat. **Read that again**. She never drew blood work, and after some arm twisting, gave me some pain medicine that only took the edge off. Around midnight, they decided to do an emergency endoscopy but found nothing, so they were discharging me. My record claimed: **patient has no abdominal pain**. The abdominal pain was why I was there. They never did any blood work, and every time I hit the button for help a tech would come in and say they would tell my nurse. But nobody came.

Around 1 am, I got up to go to the bathroom. Thankfully, they had a tech with me, because I apparently passed out. I woke up with about 5 nurses around me, IVs on each side flooding my body with saline because my BP was 70/30. I was dying, and they were discharging me. The papers were already written up. At this point, the PA decided, *hmmm maybe there really is something wrong*, and did a blood draw.

A hospitalist was called to my bedside along with a GI consult. After a blood draw, they found me severely anemic, suspected a GI bleed, and admitted me. The next afternoon, I got a CAT scan and, very soon after, found about 10 different doctors and nurses in my room. The first doctor told me he had bad news: I was going to need some kind of treatment, but at this time they really did not know what was wrong with me except the suspected internal bleeding. I was in a lot of pain and morphine wasn't touching it.

After a couple more conversations, a trauma surgeon came in, took one look at me, and it was like something out of *Grey's Anatomy*. They were running with me to the operating room, putting the cap on my head and multiple IVs in my arms while literally sprinting down the hall. I couldn't call my family and was really at the mercy of the skill of this group of surgeons. The good news is they fixed me, and I woke up in ICU a day later. The bad news is if I hadn't passed out, I was being sent home and probably would not have woken up because my counts were so low. They said, and I quote, that I was "hours from dying."

This book is not about my medical issues in general, but unfortunately, given the sign of the times, patient advocacy is now more important than it was ten years ago. If you are visiting your loved one for a couple hours a day, you become a part of the healthcare team. The only difference is that you are not on their payroll.

Good family advocacy is critical to any healthcare team. Given the current pandemic and pandemic hangover, healthcare is a bit scary. They have fewer nurses, less seasoned staff, are overworked and burned out, and it's only getting worse. The rigid pandemic visitation rules (although they are trying to reduce infection) hurts the clinical team because they mean fewer eyes on the patient. How many times have you been visiting a loved one in the hospital and had to go to the nursing station or speak to a doctor because of something you noticed that was important to their care?

I'm alive today because I was lucky enough to pass out before they discharged me. During these challenging times, please find your voice. If your loved one is ill and hospitalized, do whatever you have to do to see them. Even if the rules are for a half hour a day, get there.

"This soon will pass, I hope. In any moment of decision, the best thing you can do is the right thing, the next best thing you can do is the wrong thing, and the worst thing you can do is nothing."
-Theodore Roosevelt.

I love and miss you, Ma.

Not in Vain, A Promise Kept.

CPSIA information can be obtained
at www.ICGtesting.com
Printed in the USA
LVHW071805291121
704751LV00017B/430